A New Day Dawns

A New Day Dawns

Dawns

Breaking Up
with Abuse

ERICA GLESSING, EDITOR

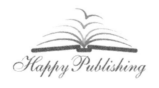

Happy Publishing

Compiled and edited by Erica Glessing

Copyright 2016 by Happy Publishing and Erica Glessing

First Edition

ISBN 978-0-9961712-6-7

Cover design by Deborah Perdue, www.IlluminationGraphics.
com

Interior design by Roseanna White Designs

"I know why the caged bird sings."
~Maya Angelou

If you receive nothing else from this book, ask yourself the question "What would it take to change this now?" and see what shows up as inspiration.

This book is dedicated to everyone, everywhere who seeks freedom from abuse. May your freedom find wings and grant you a new life you did not know was possible. Let the healing change your life, and the lives of everyone you touch, and those beyond in eight or more degrees of separation. And then what mysteries lie beyond this!

The message this book is asking once you have read it: "Please give me to a friend in need."

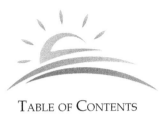

TABLE OF CONTENTS

CHAPTER 1

Kindness: The Great Wide River Flowing in You

Dr. Lisa Cooney

Constant kindness can accomplish much. As the sun makes ice melt, kindness causes misunderstanding, mistrust, and hostility to evaporate.

Albert Schweitzer

You were born to be kind – and I'm not just making this up.

According to an interview in *Scientific American* called, "Forget Survival of the Fittest: It is Kindness that Counts," kindness is 'hard-wired' into our brain.

Not that everybody defaults to it, but it's there as an innate gift.

My intention in this chapter is to shine the light on it in a way you might not have thought of before because, truly, kindness is much more than simply a good idea, or something you do to be 'nice.'

It's actually a force, or power, that, as Albert Schweitzer so elegantly phrased it, 'causes misunderstanding, mistrust, and hostility to evaporate.'

And if you have had any form of abuse in your life – past or present – you're going to want to know about this inner friend.

Personally, I didn't make friends with it until I was in my 20s, when my Family Violence professor in undergraduate school approached me one day and asked if I was okay. She'd noticed my body language, which had formed around two decades of abuse, trauma and judgment I'd lived with growing up. My shoulders were hunched up and over, nearly to my ears, in an effort to protect myself from beatings handed to me physically, verbally, and energetically.

I had other obvious kinds of behaviors, too, that came from the sexual abuse I'd endured as a child model. At least, they were obvious to the trained eye. These patterns of abuse had become internalized on many levels – both in the way I walked and held myself and in the way I communicated to myself and others.

Today, I refer to this as the 'somatics of trauma,' those ways of being that become a solidified part of our physical and energetic structure, integrated and locked in to our cellular and molecular structure.

Sounds heavy, doesn't it? Like an impregnable fortress.

Well, the good news is that, if it is, then kindness is like the siege engine that will break it down.

The Fortress of Judgment

Here's the thing about judgment…

It's been around a very long, long time – thousands and thousands of years. Humans have perfected it as a 'skill.' But that's not the worst of it.

Judgment is woven into the fabric of our DNA. We inherit it when we're born into the collective consciousness, generational lines of it that get carried down through time and passed to us. That is, until someone breaks the cycle. It's that 'sins of the father' thing.

So what does it take to break the cycle? Excellent question...

But before we do that, let's look at what judgment perpetuates in your life *if you don't*.

Judgment keeps you lying to you and locks you back into an 'invisible cage of abuse'. This keeps you locked away from you, from others, from living and certainly from creating the life you desire.

Judgment is a form of constriction and limitation, a self-destructive device and a pervasive form of *self-abuse*. It's the opposite of expansion that keeps you small and struggling, victim-like and powerless, armored and numb. As a result, you stop generating and creating beyond the cage; instead, you perpetrate you and keep the abuse cycle going.

When you judge yourself, you become your own eternal jailer and further lock yourself into the wrongness of you. Judgment returns you to the comfort of what you know (how "bad" you are) and guarantees that you never have to be more than you are right now. It solidifies the invisible cage of abuse.

When you judge another, you're actually defending, disconnecting, denying and dissociating from what you're not willing to see about yourself. I call these the '4 D's.' By design, it isolates and separates you, the opposite of oneness and belonging.

Judgment is actually something I call 'forced receiving' because, in essence, you're forcing yourself to accept someone else's judgments, particularly where you have been abused and had to receive something you didn't want – that you were forced to receive. As a result, you develop sharp, arrow-like 'quills,' like a porcupine, that can and will repel people from getting too close.

Judgments are resistances to reality that we use to protect ourselves. Many of them we learned as children either because we saw them or heard them, or because we decided them in reaction to something happening to us. These decisions then became habits of thought, the lens we see through and live by on autopilot for the rest of the flight.

The problem is that, by continuing to use them in our daily encounters with life, we cut off any other possibility we might otherwise be, do or have.

And it's to this end – clearing and transforming these judgments in order to live a freely joyful life – that I have spent the majority of my career and healing practice.

In fact, I have a name for it. I call it living your ROAR – a Radically, Orgasmically, Alive Reality. How does it get any better than that?

You're All Possibility

Your true nature is unbounded creativity, abundance, and expansion.

When you're sitting behind a desk in a cubbyhole it may not feel that way, so the best way I know to really appreciate and grow in your awareness of this knowledge is by hanging out in nature more often.

You don't even have to do anything...

It will come to you intuitively.

One of the reasons being in nature is so powerful is that the earth is the one place where judgment can't reside. It's the place you can return to again and again to release your judgments and feel the peace and possibilities of expansion. It's actually a kindness to gift your judgments to the earth.

By gifting the manure of your judgments to the earth, you literally fertilize a new possibility for yourself and everyone else.

So what is possible?

For one thing, once you let yourself out of the cage of abuse that keeps you in a 'victim' story, the whole world's wide open to you. Out there in the wild open space, you realize you have other choices for how to live and relate to yourself and others.

For example, in my case, when I discovered who I actually was beyond a shutdown, miserable, self-destructive girl, I learned I was kind, brilliant, phenomenal and funny.

Who and what is waiting to be seen by you?

As you exercise new choices, you begin to grow more confident. The old patterns of abuse no longer have power over you. You now have the power over your abuse and, with that, the power to choose a new life for yourself.

You no longer create your life from destruction, but from choice.

I know that may seem like a tall order because, quite frankly, you may be more committed to the victim story than the possibility of life beyond it. I see this time and time again in people when they first come to see me. You may feel like a victim of circumstance, as I did for so long, like there's nothing you can do to change it.

But it's a lie...

Plain and simple.

Kindness as a Generative Energy

It's common for children who've been abused to believe they're bad and wrong, but it took that conversation with my Family Violence professor in undergraduate school, and her help, to realize I wasn't worthless.

This professor was the first person who ever asked me if I was okay, and this single act of kindness flooded me with the awareness of how *not* okay I was. With her support, I began to see there was something I could do to overcome my past abuse – that I could go beyond surviving, even beyond thriving, one day.

It was as though she'd passed me the secret key to unlock myself from the cage of my own abuse.

I began to see the abusive, destructive patterns I was perpetuating through reckless behavior and I committed to choosing differently. I didn't do this on my own. It was through professional support and confidential conversations that I was finally able to release the victim story I had been living for nearly three decades.

When I let go of that, the invisible cage began to crumble away, too. I no longer needed the barriers and walls I'd erected to protect myself as I slowly realized I had other choices for how I lived and how I related to myself and others.

And it all began with that single act of kindness which, indeed, caused 'misunderstanding, mistrust, and hostility to evaporate.'

Obviously, not every moment of kindness is going to do this. Kindness wears many faces. It ranges from the simplest act – like a smile – that takes no more than a second, to extravagant offerings of help. It can be random and come out of the blue or given in response to someone's needs.

In truth, it's probably more natural to you than any other approach because, as I said in the beginning, kindness is *already in you.*

You don't have to go far to find it, although when you're locked up in judgment it can seem impossible to access. So, if you're having a hard time being kind, begin looking around for the underlying judgments blocking the view.

One way to do this is asking questions like these:

"Am I being judgment or kindness with this?" – *whether it's in relationship to money, relationship, your body, or something else.*

"Does this feel expansive or restrictive?"

"Does this feel light or heavy?"

By committing to you and accepting kindness for yourself – from yourself and others – a new space of energy and consciousness can show up – a place of receiving that is at once vibrant, alive, potent, juicy and all *deliciously you.*

Kindness ushers in a peak vitality that only requires four things, which I call the '4 E's':

Embrace what's true for you

Examine what you are actually looking at

Expand into a new possibility, awareness, and kindness

Embody the change and the truth of you

In a very real way, learning kindness is like learning a new language. In my own case, it was not a language I was familiar with. It wasn't my 'first' language, the one I heard and spoke at home. And it took practicing over time to not only learn it, but to then become fluent in it.

And, like language, it is a creating, generative energy – exactly what it takes to create a new life filled with the energy of expansion.

The beautiful thing is that, by giving up judgments and harnessing the power of kindness and gentleness, you can dissolve all the uncaring ways that you've experienced and let go of the need to protect yourself.

You can finally shed the quills and be open to receiving bountiful life – to truly be the gift you are for yourself and the world. In this place of no barriers, you will discover a softer, more vulnerable space…at once sacred and safe.

It is here that the energy of receiving flows free and easy like a great river.

You only need choose it, step into it and let it move you along its wide and generous path.

It's all yours… simply for the choosing.

Will you now?

[Source: www.scientificamerican.com/article/kindness-emotions-psychology]

ABOUT THE AUTHOR

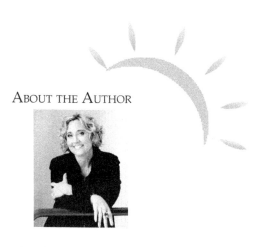

Dr. Lisa Cooney

Dr. Lisa Cooney, licensed Marriage and Family Therapist, Master Theta Healer, certified Access Consciousness Facilitator, is the creator of *Live Your ROAR! Be You! Beyond Anything! Creating Magic!*

An internationally recognized expert and #1 international bestselling author, Dr. Lisa brings an *"I'm Having It! ...No Matter What!"* approach to everything she does and teaches people how to playfully engage this magical and generative energy for creating a life that's light and right and fun for them.

Having transformed her own life from abuse and loss to a virtual playground of wonder and joy, Dr. Lisa generously shares her gifts and creative tools for transformation. She invites and guides others beyond all obstacles into a place of their own knowing... that space where they have direct access to the whisperings of consciousness.

"Are you ready to ROAR – to live your own Radical Orgasmic Alive Reality –Beyond Anything you've ever imagined?"

To contact her or to learn more about Live Your ROAR, LLC: http://drlisacooney.com/about-dr-lisa/.

CHAPTER 2

The Footprint On My Face

Sara Flowers

"What happened Ma'am?" the police officer asked me as I sat shaking in my wrecked car on the wrong side of the road. "I don't know Officer, I just lost control," I whispered through the sobs. "Are you sure you're okay?" he asked. "Yes Sir", I replied – this time more directly. "Okay, good – now are you ready to tell me what REALLY happened?" he asked again. I repeated softly, "I just lost control." Then he looked me directly in the eyes and sternly said, "Ma'am – you have a footprint on your face."

You would have thought that was my lowest point that day, sitting in the car that I wrecked because my boyfriend kicked me in the face as I was driving. Then he jumped out of the car and ran away as he left me there alone in shock, still seeing stars as the police arrived. Unfortunately, though, it was not. It was the first of many low points that I would experience at the hands of that man. The next low point was when he threatened me with a knife. I finally worked up the nerve to call the cops... only to end up taking classes for weeks to get him out of jail.

But the absolute lowest point, my rock bottom to this very day, was when I held my dead, cold infant son in my hands. I begged and pleaded for someone in the hospital room to please fix him... to bring him back... even though he had passed away the day before. He had been refrigerated since then while they waited for me to recover enough to hold him to say goodbye. Somehow I still distinctly remember several family members leaving the room, unable to "hold it together".

How did I end up there? When I was seven months pregnant, my boyfriend and I got in another fight – a fight that resulted in an emergency C-section that was too late... too late to save my son whose heartbeat was just a faint murmur for less than 20 minutes until he was officially pronounced dead. I wish more than anything that I could say this is where I left him – but it was not. That's hard to believe as I write this. I went home with him and while I still had staples in my stomach, he pushed me to the ground and ripped them out. That was the last day I saw him - although he called for weeks leaving messages and even threatening suicide until I changed my number.

As I sit here now writing this all these years later – I feel so ashamed and embarrassed to share this. I feel like I will be judged as a woman so foolish, so weak and so pathetic that it cost me my own son's life. I feel like my own innocent son paid the ultimate price for my mistakes. Then when I feel like I can't feel any lower, the thought creeps in, "Thank God I don't share a child with that man." And that is the rock bottom of my shame and guilt. But all of my shame and guilt and embarrassment is worth enduring if my story saves just one life. If just one person gets out before it gets any worse, if just one person gets away before it cost a life – then I will shout my story from the rooftops no matter what judgments someone makes about me and my choices and the life I've lived up until this very moment.

My stepdad at the time had also lost a son, so I had a confidant that knew what it was like to bury your child instead of having your child bury you. He was there as I picked out a teeny tiny white coffin – the second worst image burned into my brain. The first is that of my blue, lifeless son, of course. I had someone to talk to that really understood and knew what to say and what not to say. And then he sat down to the table during the holidays and wrote a note, took a bottle of pills and climbed into bed with my mom for the last time. She woke up and called 911 and they had her start CPR and mouth-to-mouth resuscitation until they arrived – only to realize that he was already cold. That was the day I thought I had zero chance of surviving. If this strong, fun, wise man, with a thriving business and surviving healthy son, couldn't live with the loss of his child - how would I ever make it?

But obviously I did make it. As I sit here today, I'm the healthiest I've ever been as I inspire, support and motivate others which is the ultimate reward in this life - in my humble opinion. I may not have been equipped to save my son's life all those years ago, but I'm more than qualified to speak my truth in hopes that it will help someone else. I paid in blood, sweat, tears and the ultimate loss and I hope that my debts can save someone else before they have to pay so dearly.

When I started having chest pains 6 months after my son died, I went to the doctor for an EKG that revealed I was having panic attacks which was quite understandable considering the recent events. A psychiatrist tried over a dozen medications over a six-month period, but I had such severe side effects to all of them, including insanely long periods of insomnia (that I wouldn't wish upon my worst enemy). Since my body wasn't accepting the pills, I was forced to accept the fact that I would have to make my way through this pain without numbing out. That was the beginning of my healing health journey that I continue to follow to this day. I had the body of a woman that had endured an emergency C-section (not to be confused with a standard one which has a different incision – meaning I could never have a natural birth) yet I had no child. When I was out running an errand just a few weeks after the surgery, someone asked me when I was due. I still remember how much that stung to hear as I simply walked away unable to mutter a single word or sound. That was even worse than some of the insensitive, ignorant comments that are so common. "Well at least he wasn't older." Yes, I'd much rather have no time with my child than any amount of time with my child. "Well at least you can have another one." Yes – children are easily replaced. The list goes on. I learned a valuable lesson in those experiences as well – when you don't know what to say – don't say anything at all. Or keep it to a minimal, "I'm here for you."

So here I was, young and single with a huge scar across my abdomen and an even bigger scar on my heart. But I also had love in my heart – so much love.

I've always been a sensitive person who feels very deeply for others in need. As I was growing up, my Mom always made volunteer work part of our lives. Our garage was a drop off center one year for several families in need during the holidays. We went to nursing homes, and the special Olympics and did what we could do despite never having a lot ourselves. That was until my parents got divorced when I turned 16. Due to several turn of events, I spent some time in the foreclosed home by myself and then I stayed with a boyfriend and his Mom for a while until he got in a severe car accident that left him seriously disabled. I had to leave and moved in with a female friend where I met the abusive man I ended up having (and losing) the child with.

Looking back now – I see so many patterns. I think self-awareness is the first step but that you also have to be careful not to get stuck in the stories of the past in order to create a new, improved future. So that's what I did. Way too soon after the loss of my son, I met a kind strong man who also happened to have both legs amputated above the knee. He had been an all-state basketball player who was given a full scholarship to a division one university. Just two weeks before the semester started, he was in the backseat of a car that was involved in an accident. His two family members in the front seat died while he was partially ejected. The last thing he remembers is hearing the EMS personnel putting him on the stretcher saying, "Catch his left leg – it's falling off." By the time he woke up weeks later, gangrene had spread and he had endured 4 amputations to save the top portion of his legs. He was someone who also had scars and knew pain and overcame it. He was also a man who could never kick me in the face, but it wasn't until years later (and a lot of "self-work") that I consciously made that realization.

I dated him for two years and we were married for ten. We share an amazing son together that is perfect in every way but getting him here safely wasn't so easy. When I was seven months pregnant (at almost the exact moment of my first pregnancy), my body began to show severe signs of distress. I was on bed rest with a blood pressure machine when it rose so high I began seeing stars. That's when they decided to take me by helicopter to a special neo-natal hospital where I had another emergency C-section. Although my son was two months early and weighed just three pounds, he was a miraculous fighter from day one. They told us to expect him to be in ICU in his little incubator until his due date, but he was healthy enough to leave in just 2 weeks. As I write this, he is 16 years old, around 6 ft. 3 inches tall and about to be in a size 14 shoe, so it's safe to say he has made a complete recovery. We both almost lost our lives that day and the doctor told me I should never get pregnant again.

I share these intimate moments with you to paint a full picture of how something like this can happen and how wide-spread the impact can be. While my "story" makes it somewhat easier to understand how I ended up where I did, I'm here to tell you that one does not equal the other, and that a particular beginning or even a current situation does not have to have the same ending. We both know that the chances of an abusive situation ending happily ever after are practically zero, so the real question is what price are you going to pay until you can't pay anymore? Rather than paying the price of another lie to a friend about a bruise or much worse, the payoff is practically guaranteed to be better to pay the price it takes to pick up the pieces, get out of the abuse and put yourself back together. I'm not going to lie and say it's easy but I can promise you that it's easier than staying, even though that may seem nearly impossible to believe.

I turn 40 in a few months and I consciously create the life of my dreams each day. Because of my PTSD symptoms, I was forced to create work from home which also allowed me to homeschool my son. I just spoke in San Diego last week to over 300 business owners and almost 40 joined the one-year mastermind program that I run. Because of my health issues (anemia, hypoglycemia, insulin resistance, adrenal fatigue, severe allergies, irritable bowel syndrome, anxiety, etc.), I spent years becoming a Digestive Health Specialist, Certified Practitioner of Natural Health, and a Registered Yoga Teacher certified in Trauma Release Exercises. My custom health programs radically change the lives of my clients and to see their faces when the lab tests reveal the results is one of the best feelings in the world. I am the healthiest I have ever been without one medication and I am a shining ray of light everywhere I go. Dear One – I do NOT say these things to brag because I am as ordinary and as a special as every other person on this planet. I speak these truths through streaming tears to give you hope if you need it. Wherever you are as you read this, I am a light in your life simply because I am proof that you are too. A wounded person can shine brighter than any being on the planet because they had to in order to get out of the depths of such an incredible darkness.

I have stumbled and will continue to do so but I keep choosing to move towards the light, day by day and sometimes moment by moment. I invested in myself any way I could until I finally put myself first. Once that happened, I learned a self-love that I didn't know was possible. And then the true magic happened and keeps unfolding to this very moment (and true honor) where I was invited to write to you. I blossomed into a thriving flower that could help others, after a lifetime of feeling like I couldn't even help myself. I was the mom that couldn't even protect my own unborn child and now I'm the woman who holds space for the thousands that I reach and serve. Everything that is in me is in you. I hold my hand on my heart now as I feel true love for you. I don't know when my next stumble will be although I'm certain there will be many. I do know that I will get up and keep moving towards the light. And I know that I could not do it without so many other lights like you and the incredible friends and community that I consciously surround myself with and bare my soul to. I believe in you as much as I believe in me and it is an honor to share this time and space with you as we each choose our next step towards the light together. Namaste'.

About the Author

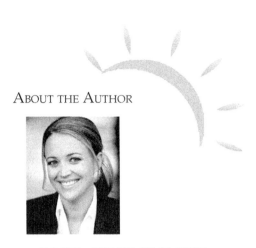

Sara Flowers – LDHS, CPNH, RYT, TRE

Sara Flowers is a health strategist for busy, stressed out women and a business consultant for 7-figure business owners and entrepreneurs.

As a Digestive Health Specialist and Certified Practitioner of Natural Health, Sara designs personalized health programs aimed at uncovering the root sources of stress that continue to sabotage most health goals. She uses a variety of professional tests and comprehensive tools in an effort to provide quick relief from health challenges related to: stress, anxiety, sleep, digestion, skin, hormones, pain, discomfort and much more.

As a business consultant, Sara designs systems to sustain and support massive growth while identifying and accomplishing other specific goals. She's helped an author and entrepreneur gross 500k/month for years in digital sales, helped a health coach create and launch a 90-day program that grossed $250K and supported a business owner with a product launch that grossed almost $4 million in less than 30 days.

Sara has spoken on stage to hundreds, made numerous television appearances, and she's the founder of the Witty Women Forum. When she's not serving clients, she enjoys a variety of dance classes, shopping at the local farmers' markets and being a Mom. Her volunteer passions incl. teaching yoga at the women's homeless shelter and T.R.E. (Tension & Trauma Release Exercises) to veterans.

For additional support, get instant access to your free copy of Sara's book at www.NourishYouNowBook.com.

CHAPTER 3

Journey Into the Light

Linda Wasil

As I wake up next to my caring and loving fiancé, I'm so, so grateful to be in this place of peace, joy and wonder. In this space, there is kindness, gratitude and the immense joy of being alive. There is not even the tiniest bit of worry, fear or fret. Only this incredible sense of knowing how magnificent a being I am. This amazing sense of gratitude that everything that has occurred in my life thus far has prepared me for this moment. And, that everything that has occurred in my life thus far has prepared me for my life's work. Everything. Period. No if's, and's or but's about it. Wow.

As I sit here and take a deep breath - I am truly amazed. Not even a second of self-doubt. Not even a nano-second. Really? Can this even be true? Holy moly, I used to be filled to the brim with self-doubt, self-hatred, anger, worry, fear and judgment. Now, there is this immense space filled with peace that my being occupies that stretches out so far around me that I can ask to continue to expand out and fill more space and more and more and more. This space gently nudges the moon, stars, gal-

29

axies, oceans, the earth, plants, wildlife and every living being. It gently washes over everything with this space of kindness and caring that is amazingly gentle yet potent. This energy wakes up and tickles the molecules of everything and everyone. This is a miracle and this is who I "be". As I bask in all of this awareness, I am so grateful for my journey....

A major turning point in my life came on June 17, 1994. When I got home from work that day I turned on the TV and watched in wonder as a white Ford Bronco was being chased by a swarm of police cars down the Los Angeles Freeway. What the heck was this? Little did I know at the time that millions were also watching and that this was the beginning of the OJ Simpson drama.

I was glued to the TV that night watching every second as the drama unfolded. As the details of that event began to air, I felt numb with the news. How could this have happened? OJ was a famous football and TV celebrity. I had watched him in the Hertz Rent a Car commercials and thought he was so charming and talented. How did this event occur with two seemingly successful people that had it all? These were people with fame, wealth and celebrity status.

Then the questions began to come. Was OJ involved with the murders and in what way? Was my situation as bad as Nichol's? Could this possibly happen to me? I reluctantly began to question my present relationship. Yes, there were signs of things escalating. I didn't want to see how things had intensified over the last few months. But, was it really that bad? I made excuses. It was difficult to look at and I went from denial to looking at a speck of truth to denial again. This cycle continued for several weeks that turned into months. Somehow, as the pieces of what occurred that night in Brentwood began to unfold, I knew that I better address what was going on in my relationship. Somehow, I couldn't hide the truth from myself anymore. I knew that I needed to really look at this even though it was extremely difficult.

And so, the process began. I picked up a pamphlet and started reading about the signs of domestic abuse. Check, check, check and check. Pretty much all of the boxes on the list were checked. Really? Basically, I had them all. Really? How had I not known that? I started to read more on the internet and eventually called into a local domestic abuse hotline and spoke with a counselor. After calling in several times, they suggested that I come into the local office and speak with someone. At first, I didn't want to come in because I wanted to keep this hidden. I was ashamed that I was in this situation and now they would be able to put a face to the voice they had heard on the phone. It would also mean that I would have to expose something that I had kept hidden from myself. I would have to actually admit that I needed help and that I couldn't move forward alone. This was a biggie for me. I basically had done most things alone and hadn't relied on anyone for help. My adage was, if I could do things by myself, then why would I need anyone else?

I continued my research and as coverage of the events of the OJ investigation continued to unfold, I couldn't avoid the inevitable. I would really need help to get through this. I realized that as much as I wanted to figure this out on my own, I couldn't. I had tried and tried and tried. I thought about different scenarios of how I was going to break up with my boyfriend. Somehow, every time I was going to get up the courage, I would back down.

That changed one rainy afternoon. My boyfriend got upset with me because I disagreed with him about plans for lunch. We were not discussing an important or life-changing decision such as buying a house, changing jobs or moving. It was something as simple as discussing where we wanted to go for lunch.

When I disagreed with my boyfriend's suggestion, he got so

upset that he grabbed my elbow and as his anger intensified, he started squeezing harder and started to twist my arm. I heard a snap and I pleaded for him to let go as the pain was unbearable. I started crying and then I yelled "STOP!" as I held my arm in pain. He finally let go. In that moment he actually had a smirk on his face. As if he enjoyed hurting me. He didn't seem sorry nor did he apologize sincerely. He just said I was overreacting and that if I hadn't been so difficult and had agreed with his plans, then this wouldn't have happened. Again, it was my fault. It was always my fault. This time I didn't doubt myself. I couldn't believe what I was hearing as anger filled up inside of me. He was actually still blaming me. For what? For not agreeing to go to lunch with him to his favorite restaurant?

This time, I spoke back and said that he shouldn't have done this and that he hurt my arm. Finally, in a sarcastic tone he apologized and said that this would never happen again. He had that familiar smirk on his face and I knew that he was lying. He wasn't sorry – he was never sorry and his behavior was becoming increasingly violent.

I decided to leave and on the 35-minute drive home, there were moments from earlier that afternoon that went through my head like a movie. I keep replaying it and replaying it trying to make sense of it. I couldn't and it was driving me crazy. There was no logic to this. My arm was throbbing and ice helped ease the pain. I couldn't sleep that night as I tossed and turned. The events of the afternoon continued to race through my mind as I keep asking myself if this was how I wanted to live my life? As I sat crying in the middle of my living room at 3 a.m., I knew that things had to change between my boyfriend and me. But more importantly, I had to get help.

By morning, I decided I needed to take the next step. I would call on Monday and set an appointment with a counselor at the domestic violence center. The hardest part was that I wanted to keep this secret. I didn't want anyone else to know what was going on.

I actually arrived at my appointment early and sat in my car under the branches of a large pine tree. I was talking myself out of getting help again. Saying that I could handle things alone and that I could end the relationship without help. It's amazing how I could so easily dismiss what had occurred the past Saturday afternoon. In that moment it was as if my arm was screaming "yes, you are going in and getting help" as the pain started to intensify again. As I held my arm, I couldn't deny the pain and what caused the pain any longer. I arrived at the appointment in a large hoodie covering my hair and sunglasses hoping that no one would recognize me. Yes, this was me, Linda, the person that had called the hotline numerous times. I needed help!

Taking this first step was the hardest. As I waited for my counselor to arrive, I started weeping. During the first session I mostly cried through a few, brief words. I actually went through a whole box of tissues and my nose was raw.

She asked me what was going on and what lead me to coming in. I told her about the incident from the previous weekend and she nodded as if this was a familiar story. There was no judgment in her universe, only kindness and caring. She said that she understood and that I shouldn't make myself wrong for what had occurred. That kept ringing in my ears – "you are not wrong Linda, you are not wrong and you have nothing to be ashamed of."

After my third session, the counselor suggested that I attend the weekly support group held in the office. She said that it would be a major part of my healing to hear what other women in a similar situation had to say. I trusted that she had my back and I was curious to meet and hear other women's stories and their healing process. What I listened to and saw stunned me.

The room was full to the brim. There were women of all ages, ethnicities and backgrounds from grandmothers to teenagers. Some barely spoke English, some were scientists, doctors and lawyers. There was even an acclaimed actress in our group and a woman that was in hiding as her abuser was about to be released from prison. This entirely blew my mind. There were so many women going through similar situations no matter what their circumstance in life. If you saw any of these women on the street you would just think they were living a normal life.

I guess I had an idea that it was mostly women from poorer families. No, I was absolutely wrong!! There were women with degrees from prestigious universities who were CEO's and founders of companies. They grew up in a life of privilege and wealth. There were also women with no means to support themselves with children that were trying to find their way.

Hearing their stories of courage and hope was incredibly healing for me. As we all spoke going around the circle, I realized we were all the same. There really wasn't a difference among us. We were all finding our way regardless of our circumstances. We all found strength and hope from each other. There was support and encouragement and everyone was able to say what was on their mind and not be judged. This was incredibly healing. Each woman had touched me in a way that was very special. We all hugged and expressed gratitude for each other. I wasn't sure if I would see any of them again in the group, however, I was stuck by their vulnerability and immense courage.

I recall returning home after the first meeting incredibly energized. Finally, I felt heard and received without judgment. I realized that I was not alone and that it actually was a strength to realize that I could receive help when it is required. It was not a wrongness to receive help. That was a huge change.

After that first support group meeting, I started to view everything differently. I didn't judge people the same way anymore.

I started to look at the energy below the surface and to be aware of what was really going on. And, I realized that I could never really know what was going on in someone's life. That was a game-changer. I had actually viewed people with money, good jobs and big houses as having it all. Now, I had a completely different point of view. Unless I was in their shoes, I really didn't know what was going on.

I continued to attend the support group and spent less and less time with my boyfriend. I lied and said I was working long hours and went away on the weekends to visit a friend or took road trips for the day. He would call constantly and at first I couldn't resist answering. After a while, I started ignoring his calls. That's when I really knew that the pull to spend time with him was weakening. I was getting stronger and reveling in all of the awarenesses.

I started to take care of myself by taking walks in nature, drawing and doing things that were fun. I attended as many personal development classes as I could and read the latest healing techniques. I studied TM meditation to help quiet my mind. Slowly, I began to have awarenesses of how I got to this point in my life...

I began to realize there were signs that I ignored in this relationship. For instance, the first time that I went over to my boyfriend's house, my body froze. It was as if I couldn't move. I didn't listen to what my body was telling me. I ignored it and thought it must be because I was nervous being over there.

When we first began dating it was all romance. Flowers, presents, home-cooked dinners, numerous phone calls and picnics on the beach. I had never been treated quite like this before and I felt special. There were promises of trips together as he told me how special I was.

At first, I discounted the many non-verbal clues. He made faces and gestures of disapproval. It was the subtle clues that over time became more noticeable. These turned into verbal jabs like – "you shouldn't eat that or you'll gain weight" or "that isn't good for you". "You shouldn't wear that – I don't like that." I thought he was truly concerned for me in the beginning... now I knew that he was just controlling me.

The gestures turned into a light slap to pinching that left bruises or tickling me until it hurt. The pieces started to come together of how slowly over time my self-esteem had eroded. And, I could see the progression of how that rainy afternoon with my bruised arm occurred.

With a support plan in place, I broke up with my boyfriend.

The healing process lasted years. I didn't date for a couple years because I didn't trust that I could choose a healthy relationship. Finally, as I began to trust myself again, I took baby steps. I started to go to parties and singles dinner events. I met a lot of men over coffee and by taking things slow while dating, I was able to see patterns of where things weren't working early on.

As I continued to cherish myself, I was attracting different kinds of men - men who listened and were kind and caring. These were men I would have discounted before because there wasn't this energetic pull or sexual attraction to them. I was opening up to relationships that had a sense of joy, ease and space. This felt so unfamiliar at first since I was so used to turmoil and upset in relationships. Slowly, kindness and caring became the norm as my gratitude for myself grew and grew. I also began acknowledging myself for the immense courage it took to get to this point in my healing process.

And now, I'm so happy to be planning my wedding to my playmate Adam. We have been dating for over six years and have so much fun together. Every day is greater than the last as we continue to explore. So much joy, kindness and caring. What else is possible? I wonder what miracles await?

About the Author

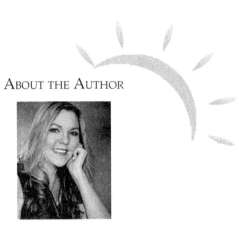

Linda Wasil

#1 international bestselling author Linda Wasil, CFMW, is a coach, intuitive counselor, author, body worker and speaker. She has always been a seeker and has studied a wide variety of healing techniques including Reiki, Healing Touch, EFT, TM meditation and countless others. However, in her practice today, Linda primarily uses tools from the body of work known as Access Consciousness™. She is a Certified Facilitator of Access Consciousness™, Certified Access Bars Facilitator™ and an Access Body Process Facilitator™.

For over 16 years, Linda has facilitated clients all over the world in living their dream of a happier, more fulfilling life through individual sessions, workshops and presentations. She is the author of "Beyond the Stigma of Abuse," a provocative book that explores abuse in a totally different way. She is also a contributing author of the Amazon Bestseller "Speaking Your Truth: Volume II" and "Financially Fit Females."

Linda has specialized in working with clients with PTSD and has found that Access Bars is a very effective modality that facilitates dynamic change for those with this condition. She also utilizes a technique known as the "Abuse Hold," which facilitates the body in releasing trauma at the cellular level. Clients have reported a sense of ease and peace with their body that they haven't experienced.

Through her healing journey, Linda was introduced to the magic of healing with horses. She rescued her first horse, Misty, from Colorado and started to become aware of how Misty was facilitating her in ways that she hadn't know was possible. As their friendship blossomed, Linda began studying hands-on energy techniques with horses. She is an equine massage therapist and studied at the acclaimed Rocky Mountain School of Massage. Linda is also a Certified Facilitator of Conscious Horse, Conscious Rider™. She facilitates this class using ground-breaking techniques from Gary Douglas, the founder of Access Consciousness™. This two-day class is open to anyone interested in learning more about horses and the magic of being around horses. It explores the joy and communion with horses that is truly possible and is about putting the fun back into riding and horsemanship.

Linda also specializes in working with clients with PTSD and has found that horses facilitate a sense of space, peace and allowance that allows for dynamic change.

You can learn more about Linda at:

www.lindawasil.accessconsciousness.com
www.lindawasil.com
www.chcr.com
www.thrivingrelationship.com

Please contact her at: lindawasil@gmail.com.

"All of life comes to me with ease, joy & glory!"™

CHAPTER 4

Survivor Thriver – Living from the Heart, Not the Hurt

Svava Brooks

I can still remember where I was driving on the Interstate 5 in San Diego and about to merge onto the 8 East. I was on route back to our apartment to finish packing up my things. I was frazzled and numb. As I was driving, I asked out loud, "God, why me? Have I not been through enough in my lifetime?"

The next thing I know, I am looking over my shoulder to see if there was someone in the car with me because I did get an answer. What I heard was, "You are here for a very important reason, Svava." It was clear and it was delivered in a way that I did not even doubt what I had heard. That was all I heard but it helped to soothe my soul in this moment and I made peace with what I was I going through, at least for that moment.

About a year earlier I met him. I was new to San Diego. I transferred to go to college with some of my friends that were attending a small international university. He was charming and handsome. We worked together in catering at one of the many hotels in San Diego. I was getting a degree in hotel and restaurant management and I was waitressing at a local hotel. After a short period of working together and hanging out, we started dating. I can't say that I can even remember exactly how we decided to get married. But soon after we were married, something changed. He changed.

I quickly realized that he was not who I thought he was. He was withdrawn, shut down, hard to connect with, and controlling. He was no longer very interested in me as a person, more in the money that I earned, and though I was working two part-time jobs and going to school, he started pressuring me to getting pregnant. I was still finishing school and found myself checking to make sure he didn't spend my student loans that were earmarked for school. I was secretly taking birth control because I was not ready to have a child. All of this while he struggled with keeping a job and would work odd jobs here and there. More and more of the living expenses and payments for his car and insurance fell on me. It was clearly one-sided as far as who was contributing and supporting us, but he kept telling me that things would get better "soon."

After about a year with him, I told myself that this was it, this was as good as it was going to get. I had settled for an unhappy marriage, an unhappy life, with no end or solution in sight.

It is hard to imagine now but I had completely given up on being happy. Looking back, I am not surprised that this was what I was used to. This is what I saw in my home growing up.

It was through an intervention that things did change. I was at a party with mutual friends and one of our friends actually asked me directly if I was happy. He mentioned that I did not look happy and if I had considered the option of leaving my husband.

What?!? I was floored. I could not believe that someone actually noticed how I was feeling. And that someone could see through my act. My whole life, I had been covering up the pain, hiding my shame and the secret of what was going on at home. I was very good at hiding it and I was very good at pretending that I was fine. The other thing that really hit me hard was that I had never considered that I had a choice, that I could choose to leave. That had never been an option before.

At least not in my childhood home, watching my mom and stepfather argue. I watched my mom get pushed around by him. Back then I never could leave. I learned very early to just accept the abuse and neglect. There was no one to tell, no one to give me options, or teach me how to speak up. No one was coming and no one cared.

It was soon after this suggestion from a friend (that I could leave) that I actually talked to him. Things had gotten worse. I heard him on the phone talking to his family that lived on the east coast. He was living a double life. I knew clearly now that I was not in love with him and he was not in love with me. He loved the idea of being with me. He loved my looks and that I made him look good. And I know he needed my money. I know he liked how willing I was to pay his bills.

Because of my childhood, growing up in a home where I never felt safe at night, I had normalized living and being in risky environments. I did not see that until later, how dangerous this man truly was.

He did not hurt me physically but he could have.

When I finally decided to leave, I told him that this was not what I wanted, that we were not really communicating, connecting, being close. I told him I wanted a divorce.

This felt incredibly risky to me and I was scared. I had never asked for what I wanted like this before, but I knew I had to, now that I had become aware and had been given a choice. I knew I had to act on it now.

The night I left, to stay with some friends, he was very upset. He begged me to stay and was really struggling with my asking for a divorce. But things had gotten to the point where I was getting more and more concerned. He was going to the police academy and as a part of that program, he had received a gun. He was obsessed with it. He slept with his gun under his pillow. I was used to guns in the house growing up but what I saw with him was that he was obsessed with the power it gave him and, at the same time, the need to feel safe and protected.

A couple of days after I left him, I went back to the apartment to gather more of my things. That was when I found the note from him. He had written a note to me, saying he had given up. He was too tired to start over again.

That was it. He was gone. His gun was gone, his truck was missing, and he had not showed up for work. During the time the police searched for him, I was scared. Where was he, would he really take his life? It was hard to believe. The police found him in his truck a few weeks later. He had driven into the mountains.

I was numb for days and really did not let it sink in what had happened. It actually took me a very long time to grasp the reality of what had happened. I had asked for my freedom, I mustered up the courage to speak up, to ask for what I needed, and in return someone had taken their life. I truly did not believe it at first and for a long time after, I expected to run into him on the street. Even though I had seen the death certificate and I had been given his ashes.

That was when I asked God, "Why me? Have I not been through enough?"

What helped me find peace about this death was the belief that God brought us together for a reason, because through him, I met my husband David. David and I met when before he died, and even though we were both in committed relationships, we both at the time recognized the powerful connection and energy we felt for each other. It was different. It was not like any other attraction that I had ever felt. We did not act on it then. But we met up and started dating about a year after the death.

We have been married for 23 years now and have three beautiful kids. David is my best friend, my soulmate, and one of the reasons why I am here today sharing my story with you. It was not easy for us in the beginning but we were committed to making our marriage work. We both came from broken families with no models of good partnerships, good parenting, and we were not shown how to heal after trauma.

With David's support I started to heal from my childhood abuse and trauma. My mom was young when she had my twin sister and I. She was groomed into marriage by a charming handsome man, just like I had. I had repeated the cycle that I grew up with, in my home, as a child.

My stepfather married my mother when I was two years old. I have memories of sexual abuse as young as four years old. My stepfather was manipulative and he groomed my sister and I into silence. The sexual abuse was always loving, so it made it confusing for a little girl to be touched in a way that made the body respond but not understand what was going on. This created a war with myself. I hated my body and I felt responsible for the abuse because I loved my daddy.

It was not until I was about eight years old that I realized that this was not a normal father-daughter relationship. By that time, I started to feel terrible shame for what he had done to me and I also started to feel responsible for the abuse. As a little girl going to sleep, I would tuck my sheets around my body telling myself that I could keep him away and if I only stayed awake this time, I might be able to stop him. But I never could. I have countless memories of leaving my body. I am floating in the ceiling watching my lifeless body in my bed. Then I would wake up the next day and find myself at the breakfast table with the whole family pretending nothing had happened, doubting myself and telling myself that it was just a dream.

I am a product of domestic violence, emotional, physical, and sexual abuse. I watched my mother being pushed around and abused by the man I thought for years was my biological father. It is hard to believe that children can endure years of betrayal and emotional and physical abuse and survive. Children and adults are incredibly resilient. I know that now.

When I started my healing journey, I had been minimizing the abuse that I had suffered for years. I told myself that it was not that bad, that others had been through worse than I had. The coping mechanism of denial combined with working incredibly hard at being perfect did serve me well growing up. I hid my shame and self-hatred growing up by working hard as an athlete, model, and a good student. The worst impact was in how I thought about myself and how I treated myself. How I harmed myself was through chain smoking cigarettes, drinking, and partying. I learned very early that my value was my body and that giving access to my body would guarantee me love or attention, or so I thought.

The healing journey was hard and painful. Now over 20 years later, I am both proud and glad I did it. I did it with God's help. I could not have done it alone and I would not trade it back for anything. It was worth it, every single step was worth it, because of what I learned about myself. I am truly proud of who I am today. I am a courageous, compassionate, and kind human being. Because of what I have been through and the truth of who I am, I am now blessed with the opportunity to help others.

I was fortunate enough to find a support group to start my healing those 23 years ago. That group saved my life and my marriage. When I felt safe enough to get in touch with the truth of what had happened to me, I was able to, with the support of fellow survivors, feel the grief and work through the excruciating pain of abandonment, betrayal, and hurt. It took years and years of getting educated about the impact of abuse and trauma, how I was living my life from false beliefs about myself, and harboring painful, negative, even hateful thoughts towards myself. Because of my childhood, I had core beliefs that I was not lovable, that I was stupid and not valuable or worthy of support, friendship, self-love or good relationships. I also learned that I was a textbook example of an adult who was abused as a child. It helped to get educated to understand the impact but what was hard at times was finding the ways to heal. To find the steps to follow, the how to's, and practical things to do to restore those broken parts and to integrate the new learning into an embodied, grounded wholesome way of living.

I committed to healing myself and was motivated to get healthy. First for my kids and to figure out to how to have a good relationship with my husband. Later for myself. In my marriage, we struggled for a long time. I was scared of trusting him. I had been hurt deeply by the people that I loved and trusted the most. How could I truly trust again?

I was afraid of intimacy and for years waited for the other shoe to fall. I was certain that either my husband did not really love me or was going to leave me. It was hard on both of us and our relationship and was painful at times. It took me twelve years to learn to trust and to open up to him and let the love in.

It was during another stand-off between us that my husband said to me, "Svava, I can't feel your heart!" He was trying to tell me that I was so defensive and aloof that he did not feel heard or validated at all about what he was asking for. It was one of those turning points in our marriage. I was crushed and felt ashamed. I didn't know what he was talking about. "What do you mean, feel my heart?!" I screamed at him and cried. It felt unfair and cruel. He was asking me to do something I did not know how to do. "Show me a picture, show me a book to read on how to do that," I yelled, "I don't know what you are talking about and how to do that!!"

The good news is that I did learn and I do know how to do that today. It is actually one of the main things I teach my clients to do as I walk them through their journey out of the hurt towards living from the heart. With my constant work on my healing journey, I also learned some important tools to communicate with my husband. We learned to settle arguments, listen to each other, and compromise. After years of frustration, we finally became good friends and our marriage shifted. I am incredibly proud of my marriage and know that it healed me and my husband. It also has been a blessing to our kids. Yes, they grew up with parents that struggled with being in good relationship, but they did see how we communicated and eventually learned to love ourselves enough so that we could come together and support each other as friends and a couple. We have modeled for our kids what a good partnership looks like. We have stopped the cycle of abuse in our families. And that is a huge blessing.

After about 10 years of my healing journey, I knew I was ready to speak out. I realized that if someone had given me the words to ask for help when I was a child, I would not have suffered in silence for as long as I did. I would have asked for help. So I co-founded a non-profit and started to educate adults about how to keep their kids safe about child sexual abuse. I brought awareness to my home country Iceland, where we sent a booklet about steps adults can take to protect kids to every single home in the country. I wanted to empower people. Yes, this is a tough issue. Yes, it is hard to talk about. In talking about it, we can not only start to prevent it from happening, but also give encouragement to the millions of victims of child sexual abuse.

Today I know why I am here and I know why me! As I have spoken to thousands of adults about the issue of child sexual abuse and how to prevent it, I have shared my story and heart openly to both heal my shame and to give others permission to do so. I did not know that I had a choice all those years ago but someone told me I could choose something else in that moment. Now I pay that forward in all my work.

I know God needed me to reconnect with my truth and my heart in order to see and feel how much love there is and it was here all along. I had to visit some dark places and experience some intense grief to be able to hold a space for others that are also on this journey.

I would not trade any of it back for anything, because what I have gained is ME! I know who I am, I know what I am, I know how I serve, and I know why. I continue to educate adults on how to keep their kids safe through webinars and trainings and I am here to help others heal and see that they too can leave the hurt and live wholeheartedly from the heart. I now teach the steps that I have been taught in my one-on-one life coaching and empower fellow survivors to practice tools that will help them accept themselves and to validate the truth. I model for them what is possible and I encourage them every step of the way.

Yes, bad things happened to them but it is not who they are. They are much bigger than that. You can choose to believe that now. I choose to believe that every day now.

And remember, nothing you can say or do will make me stop loving you, and I do – more than you know. And I will always believe that you too can heal because you also are here to share your gifts and blessings with the world, we all are. And now the world needs you, and your love and light.

Blessings!

About the Author

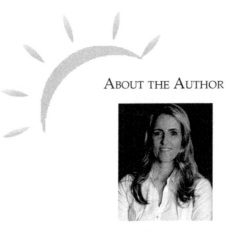

Svava Brooks

Svava Brooks is a public speaker, survivor of child sexual abuse and the co-founder of a nationwide child sexual abuse prevention and education organization in Iceland called "Blátt áfram." She is also a certified instructor and facilitator for *Darkness to Light Stewards of Children*, as well as a certified Crisis Intervention Specialist, a certified Parent Educator, a BellaNet Teen support group facilitator, and an Abuse Survivor Coach. The mother of three children, Svava has dedicated her life to ending the cycle of child sexual abuse through education, awareness, and by helping survivors heal and thrive. She is a certified facilitator for *Advance!*, a program created by Connections to restore authentic identity. Every week she writes about healing after trauma on her blog, and also leads a discussion forum on Child Sexual Abuse Healing and Recovery online.

To learn more about Svava Brooks please visit http://www.educate4change.com.

Chapter 5

Abuse Stinks

Erica Glessing

As he stood in the driveway in front of the home my mom and brother bought us, the home I gave up in the divorce, he screamed "You cunt. You whore. You slut." The kids were cowering and trying to disappear. I was in my car and I was leaving.

It wasn't like I was leaving him, then, I had left him four years before.

I am still afraid to write this chapter of my life that required so much from me to change. I am the caged bird singing, still.

I know my son is scared every time he says "I would like to go to my mom's house," when he has days over at his dad's house. He fears the anger that might erupt.

I wonder what it would be like not to be afraid.

I thought I was done with the abusive experiences that I went through when I left. I really thought I had "kicked it," and I thought I was ready to be featured in a book that helps women leave abusive relationships.

I thought if I told my story, I would give other women courage. Instead, I am not clear yet. I am still afraid. I would love to be writing this maybe 30 years from now, when I am in my mid-80s, and say, don't worry, leave, it will be alright if you leave.

Well, for me, it was better after I left. Infinitely better. And, still not alright. Not cleared. There is one person in the world who wishes me ill will. There is one person in the world who sends venomous energy whenever I am physically near him. At times, because the children aren't grown, we are in the same room or building. And then the room or building is not big enough to hold all that anger.

I didn't grow up abused, like that.

I didn't grow up with anyone laying a hand on me.

I didn't grow up in a home that was impoverished.

I chose all of that later.

I still can't quite make heads or tails of it. The experience of abuse and lies and manipulation is not something I fathom.

Before I left being married, it was not a tolerable relationship. I believe we were consuming about an 18-pack of beers daily. His co-workers would say he drank eight to nine beers before he left work most days. Most of the time we didn't sleep in the same room, he would fall asleep on the couch or in his chair in the living room.

One time he let the cigarette burn into the chair that he lived in, in the garage, and that chair burned up, nearly burning the house down.

I stood in this life with him that was intolerable, I didn't complain. I didn't stand up for me. I believe I just disappeared.

Reading these courageous stories of women who stood up, the

stories in this book, I am in awe.

I chose to stay for years, and at a huge cost. I don't know if I can quantify the cost of choices to stay "not in my body", and not rock the boat. It is painful to look at the places where I was broken and kept being broken every time I healed a little bit.

Then, I gave up material goods when I left. But I got to get me back.

The Leaving Was Joyful

The leaving was a bright moment. It was one of the brightest moments of my life. I will share that beautiful essence of my joyous bubbly self with you. It was in Los Angeles, July of 2011. I had my trio of kids, then aged about 8, 9 and 10, with me, solo, on a sports tournament trip. We were staying in a nice hotel. My room was "the best" room as we had been upgraded into a suite. So all the kids from the team came to my room, and my kids were so happy with that. There was a lot of space.

As I looked around that week, I saw all these dads who weren't drunk.

I saw all these other dads who were waking up and having breakfast with their families.

I was alone with my kids, but I was always alone with my kids. Something shifted on that trip. I saw that I could be alone, raising the kids, and it would be alright.

That trip, he showed up about five days after we did. The first night, he wet the bed. That was not uncommon. But this time, the hotel was full and they didn't have any other blankets.

So as I sat there, drenched in his urine, freezing in the air-conditioned hotel room, unable to get another blanket from the hotel management, smelling the alcohol on his breath, in that moment, I chose to divorce him.

My entire body relaxed.

My entire body laughed (although not out loud).

I didn't say anything right there on the trip. We made it back to northern California in separate cars, and I slept in the living room for a few weeks (and I took off the ring). He didn't notice.

A few weeks later he said "Is everything alright?" and by that time I had written up the divorce agreement.

In the space of the divorce, I was joyous. I lost about 50 pounds right after that, within about three months. It just fell off. It took me a long time to move out, and it took another year to wrap up the divorce, but the living hell of being with him on a daily basis was gone.

He chose to become more abusive after I left. I read about that, with the OJ Simpson case, where the man became jealous and abusive after she divorced him.

I mean, before the divorce, it was subtle and controlling, where I couldn't go out at night, and he was mean a lot. But he was also drunk a lot, and when he drank, he wasn't mean, he was kind of out of it. So maybe 80 percent of my memories of the relationship, he was out of it.

After I left him, he tried to stop drinking. Then, he became exceptionally mean. He didn't want me to go out so he would concoct all kinds of controlling reasons why I had to stay home (in my own home, not his house) with my kids.

It was like prison, basically.

It was so interesting, how people responded when I left him. My mom was dead, so she couldn't be near, and I didn't really have a lot of other family close by. I wasn't supported – not in the family, not with friends. One woman openly "shunned" my choice. I flippantly said "It is up to me whom I sleep with," only I think I said it a little differently. My kids and I stopped being invited to Halloween and Christmas events. The neighbors didn't know who to side with so we stopped being invited to NFL football games that they would watch on TV on our street.

It was an interesting time, that initial energy around the break-up. For me, I was so relieved not to have to stay in that relationship, that relief carried me through all of the social drama that was showing up. I stayed in my energy, and I stayed true, and I knew that it would all work out.

I am now in a space, five years later, where the abuse has slowed down, but it is not over.

I moved to a new home, and I found a beautiful man who treats me with kindness and respect. My new home is expansive. It spans two stories with a 400-square-foot master bedroom, three full baths, vaulted ceilings, and it has room for all of the kids and me to thrive. The back yard is so pretty and the garden is kept up.

So I'll share what worked for me to break up with the abuse that no one else could see, that I suffered silently and alone. Only even as I write this, I am clear that it is not yet over, and I am not yet free. I am afraid to write this chapter, but I'm also not willing to hold it back.

So I'm going to go through that fear into the space of helping women who may be asking for courage to leave. And also share that if your awareness is that you could be hurt, or your children could be hurt if you leave, then take different actions and precautions and you may choose to be alright with living a big lie until you can be sure you are safe, and your kids can be safe.

One of the things I found out, when I woke up and began to look around, that this "isolating" behavior is consistent with abuse. So me finding myself alone, in the abuse, was not abnormal. This might be subtle, where he doesn't approve of you spending time with your friends. Or when you do stay at dinner an extra hour, the home is in complete disarray when you return, and it's all "your" fault. Isolating behavior might be "not" allowing you to get a job or other financial means that would give you freedom to leave. It might look like caring all wrapped up in control issues.

Recognizing Abuse

The first communication I would like to share is this:

When you consider that you could be experiencing abuse, ask yourself if someone manipulates, or is unkind, or threatens, or isolates you. It is not always this huge slap or black eye or kick to your body. It could be so many different expressions of abuse, and if it is time for it to stop, you might have to be the person who stops it. In other words, you have to have your own back.

The next communication I would like to share is that there is no clear "black and white" and also, there is. So even when it doesn't seem to be perfectly clear, it often is, and we can't see it because of all the follow-up choices that show up when we are seeing the abuse with clarity. By this I mean when you do see something that is terribly wrong in your world, and you "must needs" change it, that will have repercussions. Your awareness may choose to block knowing anything, because once you do see the repercussions, this means change. Allow yourself to have awareness of abuse, and allow yourself not to act until you are ready to act – even when you see things that are horrible in your world. I'm not saying "don't act." I'm saying, allow yourself the awareness of everything without judging you, or anyone else. And then as the awareness becomes more and more clear, ask for solutions that will work out "for the best of all."

Suddenly when the veil is removed, and the behavior is seen for what it is, our whole life needs to change. And this may be daunting. So we may choose not to truly see the abuse, for in seeing it, what other choices would we have to make? I personally had to make very difficult choices – although, in retrospect, I don't believe I made any of the choices soon enough!

And it may be possible that nothing is perfectly clear. It is this very intermittent nature of abuse that makes it challenging to spot and clearly cut it out of your life. I would say to myself "He isn't always so bad."

Ask Empowering Questions

Here are some empowering questions you can ask yourself:

Would staying in this relationship the way it is now be of service to my highest expression of me?

Is it dangerous to leave?

What can I put into place to create and generate a safe way of leaving abuse?

If you are afraid to leave, know that you may be tuning into potential violent reactions to you leaving. Don't ignore your intuition. It's easy for those outside of you to say "leave already." One of my friends actually offered me an entire set of furniture if I would leave, and said I could always come and share her home, with my kids.

I'm not saying "don't leave" or "leave," I'm saying tune into your intuition and if you are getting that it could be worse after you leave, then put precautions into place.

The law doesn't always get how to help.

Your friends may not get how to help.

Society sometimes in general decides "It's better to stay

together."

So when you leave, don't look to "society" to support you.

And yet, when you are being true to you, you are changing the world for all the others, men and women alike, who are seeking the courage to break up with abuse.

Every time you honor you, you make it easier for all of the people in your world to honor themselves.

So, you matter.

Here are a few more questions you can ask yourself:

What is beautiful about me I forgot to see?

What is precious about me I never remember knowing?

When I look back to the baby I was, fresh and new in the world, what would that baby being ask for its reality now?

When I jump ahead a decade on my timeline, what would I like to see surrounding me? Let's say it is 10 years from now, and I'm looking back, what choices would my "future" me recommend I make?

If I were my own daughter, what would I wish for me to experience? What would I say to "me" as my daughter that shows up as wisdom?

There is wisdom and great love for you for all of the things you are and do. This love can express itself bigger when you are surrounding yourself with kindness. I encourage you to take chances on you. I encourage you to trust your knowing. You are the master of you.

About the Author

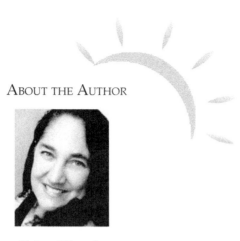

Erica Glessing

Erica Glessing is a master of happiness, creative expression, and joy. Erica began writing professionally in 1982, and won awards as a journalist in the 1980s and 1990s. She's a #1 international bestselling author 18 times over, and runs the company Happy Publishing from her home office in Northern California. She teaches happiness, and speaks and writes about happiness with a commitment to changing the vibration of consciousness on the planet. You can find her "60 Days of Happiness" at http://happypublishing.net/60-days-of-happiness-with-erica-glessing/, where you can listen to Erica share her insight into choices you can make to change your life, today. Erica is the mom of three beautiful teens and two kitties.

CHAPTER 6

That Day

Grace Hart

Hey you! Beautiful you!

I know you may not be feeling beautiful right now, and that's okay. You may be going through big stuff where you can't see a way out, and that's okay. You may feel alone, you may be scared, that's okay too. You may feel trapped, overwhelmed, hurt, betrayed, always wrong… that's understandable and it's all okay.

Why? Because from my experience I absolutely know that in spite of everything you've been through you're not alone and a different future is possible. You have the universe, consciousness, me and every other author in this book by your side. No matter what's going on for you right now or how good or bad you may be feeling, you are amazing and courageous for reading this book, for never giving up.

Things are about to change for you in magical, miraculous ways you never thought possible. How do I know? Well, because I'm magical and when I care about someone, their life gets better as if by magic! It's one of the potencies I have.

So my friend, I have your back, and I wonder what else is possible now? I wonder what your magical potencies are that you have never acknowledged? Are you ready to dive into possibilities with me? Let's go for it!

Let's start with 'that day.'

You may not remember it. You may not even be cognitively aware of it. 'That day' may have actually occurred in another space, dimension, reality, non reality, or even another lifetime. You may have hundreds, thousands, or even trillions of 'that day's.'

What is 'that day'?

That day is the day you made yourself wrong. That day is the day you chose to separate from your awareness. That day is the day you made abuse bigger than you. That day is the day you bought the lie you are wrong, alone, helpless, or a victim. That day is the day you started lying to yourself. That day is the day you gave your power to choose away. That day is the day you stopped choosing for you and started choosing against you. That day is the day you broke down and sobbed. That day is the day you hid the bruises or lied about how you received them. That day is the day you told yourself they didn't mean it, they're just really stressed, that if you just changed your behaviour, if you just cut yourself up into smaller pieces to please them, it would all be okay. The conflict would end if you could just get smaller – sooooo small no one would notice you, then it wouldn't be so bad. That day is the day you bought the lie it was all your fault, that you deserved it. That day is the day when you gave up on you. That day is when you no longer had your back or the backs of your kids. That day is the day you got you were dying inside. That day is the day your body and/or your being started to choose death.

59

The thing about 'that day' is that you have also experienced it another way. Again it may not have occurred in this lifetime, you may have experienced it in another space, time, dimension or reality. What I know for sure is you HAVE experienced this other sort of 'that day.'

How is this 'that day' diffferent? It's that day you knew that something greater was always possible.

It's that day you knew you had total choice and the ability to choose and change anything that wasn't working for you. It's that day you were adored, seen and received from a space of sweetness and kindness. It's that day when you just knew you were beauty walking, joy in motion, when you knew you were magical. It's that day you laughed, sang, and knew you were free to be all of you. It's that day when you didn't have to look over your shoulder. It's that day when someone raised their hand to swoosh a fly from their face and you didn't freeze. It's that day you were free to love another. It's that day you knew you are and have always been a gift, here to change the world.

Oh... and that day was the day you knew you were never wrong, ever... ever. You are not wrong. There is nothing wrong with you. There never was and there never will be, okay?

It's the day you knew you are a miracle walking.

Do you remember that day? How long ago was it? Can you recall it? Was it this lifetime or another?

Sweet being, can you do something for me? Allow your energy to expand out in all directions including down into the centre of the earth. Now, fill the room you're in. Great! Now expand out to fill the building you're in. Awesome. Now fill the country you're in. Cool! Now expand your energy to fill our sweet planet. You're really cool at this! Now expand further out to the galaxies and beyond...

See…how amazing are you? Did you just do that without thinking? Was it easy? And maybe even a little bit fun? Do you feel any different? Maybe lighter?

Right now think of someone or something that has bothered you or frightens you. Get the energy of it. Does it feel heavy? Constricted? How would you describe the energy? What are you aware of in your body when you think about it?

Now expand the energy baby! More, more, more… and more. Yipeeeee! Yes, yes, more, more, make it infinite! More, bigger, bigger bigger… awesome beautiful you. Now what's happened to that energy that was sticking you? Has it disappeared? How are you feeling? Better, worse, the same? Lighter? What would happen if you used this tool every time you felt yucky?

I'm about to share something that seems too easy, too magical, can't possibly change your life. I get it! I really do! A few years ago I was under the biggest pile of poo, and what was really crazy was the poo had been there for so long I thought the poo was me!

I didn't get it was just poo made up from all the mean things others had said to me – and I had said to myself – about me and my body. It was all the judgments and points of view (POV) I had created, invented, bought from others and sold to myself as real and true about me, and I gave myself the job of covering myself in the poo (making my problems and wrongness of me real) so that that's all anyone noticed. What I didn't realise is that every part of that poo was a lie!

Your POV create your reality, your reality does not create your POV! When I changed the POV of my poo being real and true – when I chose the POV that it was a lie, magic happened. The poo pile started to get smaller and smaller – as did my problems… the problems that only a few moments before seemed so solid and unchangeable.

Opportunities magically started to show up. I started to make money. Beautiful people showed up around me that did not see a pile of poo, but the beauty and gift I was to them and to our world. I started to laugh again, I started to sing. I started to have my own back, I started to have my kids' backs. I started to choose for me, not against me. I started to choose to live.

So here are the starter tools I used that changed everything for me. Tools that seem soooo easy you may think it won't work.

It was 'that day' when I chose to give these tools from Access Consciousness® a go.

1) Light and Heavy. If something feels light it's true for you, if it feels heavy it's a lie.

If I said to you, "You are a horrible person" does that feel light to you? Does it feel heavy? I'm assuming it felt heavy. Why? Because it's not true for you, it's a lie. I just lied to you and that's why you felt a heaviness and a contraction in your body. If I said to you "You are a gift" does that feel light or heavy? I'm assuming it was light and perhaps even made you smile, why? Because it's true for you! You ARE a gift! A beautiful gift... yes YOU!

If the way your partner, friend, lover or family member speaks to you feels heavy, it's a lie and not true for you. If it feels light for you, it's true for you. So when they say something to you and you catch that it's heavy just acknowledge it's not true for you. You don't say it to them, just to yourself (with your inside voice), 'Oh that's heavy. It's not true, they just lied.' ... and then use this next sentence to say bye-bye to that energy, "It's not true or real, it's a lie, bye-bye!"

If my second question felt heavy to you, that's ok... you have just made your pile of poo so real that it's true for you, and you probably have the POV (point of view) that you're not a gift. That will change when you drop the poo POV so you can receive what's true... that you're a gift.

While you're still buying some poo as true, allow me to let you know, beautiful you, right now, what's true for me... what I know for sure.

You are a gift. A beautiful, magnificent gift. This may be the first time you have been told this. I wish you would have been told this before you came into this world and every day thereafter just how amazing you are. Yes you, reading this now. You, my friend, are beautiful, special, a gift. I see it, I know it. I'm sorry for all the mean things that were ever said to you. I am so, so sorry. I'm sorry if you didn't realise until this moment that you are beauty walking and you are here to change the world.

I began by paying attention every day to how my body and being were responding to the words people said and the things I thought. If they were heavy I knew it was a lie and I'd say to myself, "You are a lie, bye bye! I'm not going to lie to myself any more." I also noticed when I or other people said things that were light, and then I would say, "Oh, I just told myself something true for me." I'd then expand that yummy energy and ask, "Please show me, consciousness, what else is possible and how does it get better than that?

2) If I choose this, what will it create?

Once I realised that if it's light it's true, I started to only choose things (people, events, parties, work, homes etc.) that matched that energy of lightness. If I was asked out or I was choosing what to eat, or I was about to say something to someone, I'd take a moment and ask, "If I say yes to this, or ask this, think this, worry about this or do this what will it create?" And then I would not look for the answer. I was actually asking to perceive the energy of what shows up when I asked the question. If it felt light I'd do it, and if it was heavy I'd say, "Oh, if I choose you I will create more poo! More wrongness, more lies, more problems, no thanks, not today!" I'm creating my life now, no longer on auto poo pilot. (Giggles.)

Hang on. Creating your life? I had no idea I could create my life. I was on auto poo pilot and my life was all about surviving and maintaining the poo (problems).

Wait a minute Grace, are you telling me I can choosing something totally different from my problems? Don't I have to fix them first? Understand them? Get over them? Get through them? Deal with them?

Well beautiful ones, the answer is no. You don't have to fix what's wrong in your life to have a greater one show up. That was a huge light bulb moment for me. I didn't have to roll around in my poo, trying to figure out why it was there, trying to figure out why more and more of it kept showing up no matter how much I looked at it, fixed it, thought about it, spoke about it, got therapy about it.

So Grace, you're saying I can just leave the 'thinking and fixing' and just choose something totally different?

Yes!

The way I freed myself and continue to create the life I choose is by not buying the lies (heavy poo poo pile) I had around me, and moment by moment followed the lightness. Without even lifting a finger (or shovel) my pile of poo (problems) sorted themselves out with ease, or just plain disappeared as if by magic. Or I'd hear something, or bump into someone who could assist, or I'd have an idea or awareness just pop in out of the blue. Without going into details, my pile of poo was impressive! Financial, emotional, health and family issues. It was a huge mess that if you knew me then you would have probably agreed that it would be impossible to change.

Held within these words of this chapter are some of the first steps and tools I used to change everything. It was 'that day' for me that I made the demand that I stop with the self-abuse. It was 'that day' I chose to live. It was 'that day' that it was no longer okay to create, choose and invite abuse into my reality. It was 'that day' I said to myself while sitting in an Access Consciousness® class, "No more, this stops now, even though I can't see a way out, even though I feel so alone, even though I feel so pathetic and wrong, this stops now!" It was 'that day' I realised that everything I said in the previous sentence was heavy – when I said, "I'm alone," it was heavy. When I said, "I am wrong and bad," it was heavy. When I said, "I can't get out or see a way out," it was heavy. That was 'that day' I got that it was all a lie and those lies were keeping the abuse in existence. It was 'that day' when I started to have my back. With each choice I made, and with each lie I said bye bye to, I became more of the beauty and magic I now know is me.

My 'that day's' are now filled with adoring, magic, wonder, travel, running classes all over the place, giggles, laughter, questions, choice, possibilities and contribution. And I keep asking what else is possible and how does it get better than that?

Beautiful ones, please know that creating a poo life is a choice. No choice is a choice. Going into the wrongness of you is a choice. Giving power to the energy of abuse or your abuser is a choice. Trying to work things out is a choice and so is choosing to make your problems more real than the gift of possibility you be and are. In every ten seconds you can choose to live on Planet Problems (that's the place where you buy all the lies that you can't change your life, where you make judgments, abuse, violence and problems true and real) or... you can fly baby! Choosing to fly is choosing Planet Possibilities (that's the place where you create your life, one choice at a time, where you are no longer functioning from auto poo pilot, where you choose and have a life of ease and joy and you function from infinite possibilities.

For me the change happened when I chose to no longer tell myself what or who I was afraid of or what could not change (or whatever else I thought the problem was). My life changed on that day... those moments I chose to speak about possibilities, to follow the lightness no matter how flickering it was. I asked the universe to show me something beautiful. I asked the universe to show me what else was possible and how does it get better than this? I did this no matter how good or bad I was feeling. Every time I asked, the universe delivered, and that's how a new life of infinite possibilities was created where this once wrong, abused pile of poo existed.

'That day' was the day I broke up with abuse.

It's a memory now... 'that day'. I still don't quite comprehend how it all changed so easily once I followed the lightness and possibilities. I don't choose to try to understand it. I just know it worked, it still works and it will work for you too!

What else is possible, beautiful you?

Universe, please show the magical being who is reading these words something beautiful today...

About the Author

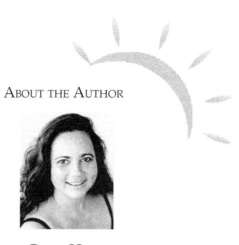

Grace Hart

Grace grew up in mainstream society, until one day a car accident in her late teens changed everything. She was rushed to hospital in a critical condition, with 48 broken bones. At the time of the accident, Grace had a near death experience and woke up incredibly aware and potently psychic.

Grace can relate to the many challenges people face, she's been "there and done that" with diverse life experiences and the associated highs and lows covering the full emotional spectrum. She has 3 children. She's been the wife of a senator, travelled the world, met many famous people, is currently a single mum, and knows what it's like to struggle and experience intense physical pain.

Grace is an experienced clairvoyant medium, and has read for famous actors and politicians. While Grace was promoting her book '*The Peacemaker's Way*', she was approached by the Dalai Lama's official bowl players, who gifted her with a set of their Tibetan singing bowls, opening up a new avenue for Grace of therapeutic sound. Grace then produced CDs of soothing, therapeutic, meditative music that is mesmerizing.

Grace has had an interesting life journey filled with many situations that led her to a point of seeking and a knowing that there HAD to be something greater than this. Through this questing Grace discovered the tools of Access Consciousness® and that has propelled Grace forward into a life of infinite possibilities and will often be heard giggling.... *"How does it get any better than this?"*

Grace is the author of *"The Peacemaker's Way"*, some of her life experience is featured in this book *"A New Day Dawns: breaking up with abuse"* and the soon-to-be-released *"The Energy of Magic"* and is currently completing *"The Victim Song"* (on domestic violence) and *"Receiving Wonderland"* (about Possibilities).

CHAPTER 7

Witness

Kaarin Alisa

When my husband came home, he was surprised to find me lounging on the couch having tea with his girlfriend. He pulled up a chair and said, "Well, I guess this was bound to happen at some point."

I was devastated… but something was different. I no longer felt alone.

For nearly five years, this man I called my husband had systematically eroded my self-confidence and isolated me from my family and friends. The abuse was mental, emotional, and physical, but worst of all; I had fallen into a place where I felt there was no way out.

But this day, when his lover knocked on my door and introduced herself, I was face to face with someone who understood completely. In her, I saw a mirror of me; accomplished, intelligent, and under the spell of someone unworthy of her love and respect. I saw a woman whose life would be so much better without the abuse. And she saw the same in me. Together we threw off the yoke of this abusive man and stood as one as we kicked him out of our lives permanently.

And while this describes one very extraordinary day in my life, had it not been for the coincidence of the day, I may have continued indefinitely to suffer the abuse he lavished on me.

I was lucky – I had found a witness!

The abuse I suffered from this man had been complete. It was systematic and calculated to wear me down to the point where I was compliant and servile. And as dramatic as it was, it taught me about abuse in ways that only living through it could.

Here is what I learned – the mind that accepts abuse, and remains servile to it, is caught in an illusion – a mind-made illusion. The illusion says that the abused is powerless, deserves the abusive treatment, or otherwise has no help, no way out, or no place to go.

Why a Witness?

Witnesses are important. However, no one can "tell" you it's wrong to allow the abuse to continue. No one can push you into changing any situation, even an abusive one. Someone who tries to order you, shame you, shun you, or guilt you into change is not a witness. A witness sees, and helps you see a sharp and accurate reflection, as if in a shiny mirror.

When you are enmeshed in an abuse cycle, it doesn't matter where the abuse is coming from. It doesn't matter how big or small its effects or how long you have been caught in the web the abuse weaves. The only thing that will help you remove the abusive situation is someone standing with you in compassion and love. Someone who says, "I understand, I know this is hard, and let's do it anyway – let's take action."

When you are inside the illusion abuse creates, everything you see, feel, and hear about the abuse, feels like a continuation of the abuse. You hear the words of loved ones through the illusion's effects. So when your best friend says, "Geez, are you ever going to change this?" it's heard as a recrimination, as a judgment. You'll take it as just one more part of the abuse cycle. When a family member says, "What's wrong with you? When are you going to stand up for yourself?" it's the same. It's just one more voice joining the abuse chorus heard from inside the illusion.

We are human, after all. And humans are adept at rationalizing and making excuses for anything we feel powerless to change. We will blissfully, or painfully, continue to rationalize out of the real and into the illusion day in and day out until something more powerful than the illusion cuts through and makes itself known. And the only thing more powerful and more real than any illusion on Earth, is genuine caring and the compassion and empowerment generated from a true expression of love.

I'm not talking about romantic love. I'm talking about the expression of love that comes directly from the heart, available to us through our divine nature. This type of love is powerful, it is larger than fear, and it is grander than experience. When expressed, this love harbors no judgment. It sees divinity equally in all beings and seeks to inspire all beings it touches to express themselves through love as well.

When this type of love touches us, our spirits rise. Our ability to cut through illusion strengthens. When this type of love touches us, we are reminded of who we are and what we deserve by the very nature of our inner divinity. This type of love is compassionate. It will see, but will not add to, anything that demeans who we are. Too often people express compassion from a place of pity, and pity is a state in which we accept the situation as just our lot. Pity condones victimization. Love in its pure form does not accept anything that diminishes; instead, it inspires us into greatness of self.

It takes a witness to be able to fulfill this role. It takes someone who can help you see the truth in a way that doesn't prompt your need to rationalize or shrink, because what you see when you look at the witness is what exists on the other side of the abuse illusion. Maybe a friend can stand with you without judgment, without recrimination, but with compassion and love instead. Maybe a therapist or a professional energy worker can do this. It may be a family member, or as in my case, a stranger that can fulfill that role.

Or – it may be yourself.

Yes, you can be your own witness.

Sometimes there is no one else but you to muster the compassion needed to break the illusion's spell. If there seems to be no one left to turn to, or if all the people around you are fed-up, angry or judging what they see in your life, there may be no one but you to stop the judgment and raise the compassion level high enough to make a difference in you.

How to be Your Own Witness

Being your own witness is possible. It may seem impossible when you are in the illusion of the abuse, but it is possible. Here is an effective 11-step process that you can do right now to lift yourself into seeing you with the eyes of a compassionate witness:

1. **Acknowledge**: First, acknowledge the abuse. If you are suffering with a situation that brings you pain, that forces you into a subservient role, or otherwise tries to convince you that you are powerless or deserving of pain and recrimination, it means you are suffering from abuse. Admit to it. You don't yet have to believe anything about yourself – your deservedness, your power, or your abilities – merely admit abuse is happening.

2. **Look in the Mirror:** While you are alone, turn off the phone and any other distraction and stand or sit in front of a mirror. Your first glimpse of yourself in the mirror may return feelings of disgust or anger or pity or any other judgmental emotion. That's okay! These emotions merely reflect how you feel from *inside* the abuse illusion.

3. **Relax:** Close your eyes and breathe deeply a few times. Let your shoulders fall well below your ears, let your jaw relax until your teeth part a little bit. Keep your eyes closed.

4. **Imagine a Friend:** Now, imagine in your mind a person who resembles you, but is not you. Imagine her in detail. Imagine that you have known her almost all your life and that you love her deeply. Give her a name.

5. **See Her Story:** Now imagine that she is suffering from the same type of abuse as you. Make it real in your mind. The abusive situation in your life mirrors the situation in her's completely. See her reflect the same disempowerment the abuse sets-up in your life.

6. **Offer Love:** Tell her that you love her, that you are ready to stand with her to stop the abuse if that is what she wants. Tell her you love her either way, even if she doesn't want to stop the abuse or isn't able to find her way out. Your love for her is unconditional.

7. **Feel Your Heart:** Now feel your heart open with this unconditional love. When you feel your heart expand in love for her, open your eyes and see her in the mirror. See her completely. Continue to extend your love to her unconditionally.

> *If, when you opened your eyes and looked in the mirror, your mind snapped back to you*

*and your own painful thoughts, merely close
your eyes and start again at step 4.*

8. **See Your Friend:** Eventually, when you open your
eyes and look in the mirror, you will see your beloved
friend looking back at you. When you see your friend in
the mirror and you feel the deep and unconditional love
you have for her, then look over her face. See from her
the same unconditional love reflect back to you with as
great a force as you love her. Know that she is willing
to stand with you as witness, even if you falter or have
difficulty finding your way. She will stand with you as
witness.

9. **See the Real and Ask:** When you see her and feel her
in this way, your eyes are temporarily able to see the *real*
instead of the abuse illusion. This is the time to ask her
what the next step is. She will tell you. The next step may
be an action that you can take right away that helps you
move toward dissolving the abusive situation. The next
step may be remembering that you do have a loved one
or a professional you can call for help. It doesn't matter
what the next step is, you can know that this action step
was given you by a friend who was looking at your situation through the real instead of through the illusion. In
this way, you can trust it.

10. **Be Grateful:** Thank your new friend for her help and
go back to your life empowered with a clear action step.

11. **Take the Action:** And as promised, take the step she
offered you.

You can perform this exercise repeatedly for each new action
step needed until you are able to see the real with regularity.
This is powerfully being your own witness.

Remote Abuse

If the abuse is coming from a remote source, perhaps coming to you telephonically, or by email or text, or if the remote abuse is coming at you energetically, as in someone sending you darts, arrows, or vibing you with anger or other abusive emotions, consider taking steps to protect and neutralize the energy from the offending party as soon as possible.

This is a good time to call a professional energy worker to set-up personal protection from the situation. Some situations can be immediately dissolved or neutralized by a good energy worker. Other situations may need temporary protections put into place while physical remedies are employed over time.

If you feel empowered to it, perform some of these quick remedies yourself, and call a professional if the steps you take are not enough to be effective in neutralizing the energy.

1. **Ask, Is this Yours?** When the energetic abuse begins, recognize it as coming from someone else. Ask yourself, 'Is what I'm feeling mine or someone else's?' If the answer is someone else, immediately send it back to where it originated. If it's not yours, you don't have to accept it or keep it.

2. **Call in Protection:** Call in your own protections. It may be God, Jesus, Angels, Archangels, Kuan Yin, Ganesh, or any other guides or masters you work with or believe in. Any of these can be called upon for immediate protection and shielding from abusive energy. Ask them to stand with you and keep you whole and free from the destructive intentions.

3. **Erect a Barrier:** Erect an energetic barrier between yourself and the sender. Some people are fond of mirrors that will continually send everything back to sender. Some prefer a bubble of energy that can discern

which energy to allow through and which to bounce off.

Remember that no matter what you or an energy worker does energetically, if the abusive behavior does not stop, take steps in the world to make it stop. This may include legal action. Each situation is unique, so determine for yourself what action is needed to get it to stop.

Freedom

Above all, remember that you are a child of the divine. Remember that any situation can change over time. If you take steps toward freedom, freedom will eventually find you.

ABOUT THE AUTHOR

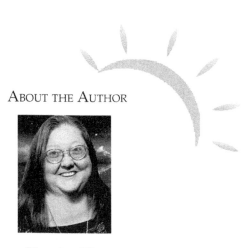

Kaarin Alisa

Kaarin Alisa is a catalyst for spiritual growth and personal transformation. She has honed her abilities as a change agent in the metaphysical and energetic arts for more than forty years, practicing as a spiritual adviser, Certified Clinical Hypnotherapist, teacher, and energy practitioner. She has helped people from all walks of life realign to their highest truth, so they are better able to pursue their dreams and ambitions.

As a child, Kaarin was blessed with intuitive vision that society tried to suppress, sometimes with painful consequences. But thanks to her burning desire to be of real service to others, she kept her intuition intact, and by the age of 15, she was giving readings and working as a psychic medium. At that time, she also began work on the *Rabika Oracle*, an uncanny divination card system. This tool took more than 20 years to develop, and can now be experienced as free online readings; soon, also to be available as a physical card set and accompanying guidebook.

Over the years, Kaarin has authored many books in diverse genre such as technology, history, self-empowerment, metaphysics, and spiritual living. Her latest bestselling book, *Bare Bones: The Unabridged Life of Yeshua son of Joseph from Galilee*, reveals Jesus' largely-misunderstood life as it was disclosed to her through her many conversations with him.

Kaarin also runs the *Goddess Speak Project,* and is in the process of developing *The Center for Conscious Choice.* Her transformational show on KCOR Digital Radio called *Consciousness Revolution* is an extension of her inner calling. Kaarin also offers classes, webinars, and private sessions by appointment.

http://kaarinalisa.com
http://rabika.com
http://barebonesbook.com
http://goddessspeakproject.com
Facebook page: kaarin.alisa.author
Twitter: @goddesses_speak

CHAPTER 8

Kindness and What It Really Means

Andrew Rigg

When I was asked to write a chapter in this book, I was amazed at the trust Erica had in me as, well, I'm a man and this is a book predominantly about women leaving abusive relationships.

Consequently, I feel totally blessed to be writing for such a book. What I'm about to write is about kindness and how people often misunderstand what kindness is. As I explore kindness, there will be some things that I mention that may create a lightbulb moment and other things that you know already. My hope with this discussion is to open the doors to a greater possibility with kindness and to recognise those people that are not kind with greater ease.

Before I go into what kindness actually is, I'd like to have a look at the pretence of kindness. The pretence of kindness is where people are kind to you to get something from you. That could be sex, money, relationship or something else. It actually doesn't matter what it is. The point is that these people use the pretence of kindness as a way to get something from you.

That, unfortunately, is not kindness; that is scoundrel. They are only using the pretence of kindness. I get it that there are many scoundrels out there so be on the watch for those that have the pretence of kindness.

Before I go any further, I'd like to explore the definition of kindness. Kindness is an Old English word, derived from *kyndnes*, that meant "nation; produce, an increase." It also meant "courtesy, noble deeds." The adjective *kind* meaning "friendly, deliberately doing good to others," is from the Old English *gecynde* meaning "natural, native, innate," originally "with the feeling of relatives for each other." With all this in mind, it's clear that the word kindness invokes feelings of contribution, gentleness and friendliness. People who are scoundrels don't operate like this. They may be gentle and friendly but they certainly don't wish to contribute to you. Scoundrels wish to control you or take from you.

Now there is another point of view about what kindness actually is. I am an Access Consciousness® Certified Facilitator and Access Consciousness® defines kindness as the ability to totally perceive another person's reality and deliver exactly what they require. When you operate from kindness, you deliver exactly what the person can actually receive. It you don't operate from kindness, what you deliver to the person may not be kind. In kindness, you know what someone can't receive and you can give him or her a seed of information that would allow him or her to receive it in the future.

Putting the dictionary and Access Consciousness® definitions together, we come up with something that allows a person to contribute to another in such a way as to allow them to receive it easily. This also includes kindness to self.

Kindness to self is where you know what you require and you do whatever it takes to do it or get it. In an abusive situation, what you would require is to get out of there. Are you willing to be kind enough to yourself and get out of the situation? Obviously, if you're reading this book, you certainly are. When you are kind to yourself, some people can misinterpret this as being selfish. Honestly, if you are in an abusive situation, does it really matter what others think? There is no one out there but you that can actually be as kind to you as you.

Another aspect of kindness is that other people can take advantage of kind people. When you are being taken advantage because you are kind, are you actually being kind to you? You might well be kind to others but, of necessity, that kindness must also be expanded to include you. If not, you will always be taken advantage of because you have missed the very essence of kindness. Kindness includes being kind to you.

Often people stay in relationships that are abusive for very varied reasons. It could be children. It could be control. It could be a whole range of things. It's not the purpose of this discussion to go into the reasons why people stay in such relationships. When you do stay there, how much kindness is there for you?

Kindness is not buying a gift for someone on his or her birthday. It's not saying the right thing at the right time. It's not taking on a responsibility for someone. Kindness is simply the ability to perceive exactly what a person requires and to deliver that and only that. You see, when you deliver something else, do people like that? No. For instance, you see a friend in need and you offer them money. They look at you and say, "do you think I'm a charity case?" Whoa! You were just being kind. Or were you? That is actually superiority in the sense that you decided what they required, you gave it, it wasn't what they were asking for and then they returned it with daggers attached. What if what they actually required was simply a hug? What if they required an income stream - not charity - and you knew someone who was looking for someone that has their skills? It's not actual money that you're giving; you are giving empowerment. You are giving them exactly what they require in the moment and nothing more. You are empowering them to make a different choice. That is kindness.

When you give someone more than what they require in the moment, that's what we call caring. Caring often comes with obligation and it often comes from the point of view of "I know what's best for you." I'm sorry, as I said earlier, that is superiority. Sure, you may know what is best for them but it is their life and they need to live it as they choose. If they continue to choose people who are abusive, then only they can choose a different type of person. You can't do it for them. You can't tell them that the person they are with is abusive until they are ready to hear it. Choosing to tell them before they are ready to hear it is not kind. Choosing to wait until they are ready is a kindness; it's a kindness to you as if they are not ready, they will fight you to prove that they have made the right choice. Remember kindness includes being kind to you.

Now, let me talk a little about contribution. Often people misconstrue contribution as only giving money. Yes, that is a contribution but it is only one type of contribution. A contribution can be a hug, a shoulder to cry on, having a meal with someone, or simply spending time with him or her. It is actually something that gives the person a sense of peace and space in order to make a different choice, if they choose. They don't have to make a different choice, you are simply giving them the possibility to make a choice, which they feel they cannot do on their own, and you are also letting them know that you are there for them. You effectively "have the person's back".

Having someone's back is also a part of kindness. When someone has your back, they are there for you no matter what happens. They are there to support you in the best of situations and the worst of situations. They are also there to tell you, "hey, that was a stupid thing to do." Telling you that it was a stupid thing to do is also support in that they are looking out for you. They know that if you continue to do this thing, whatever it is, you are not going to end up in a happy place. They know that it is your choice and regardless of the choice you make, they will be there for you and they will not make you wrong for the choice you make. They may not be around all the time but they are the person that not matter what occurs, they are there for you. The important part here is not making you wrong for the choice you make. A person that truly has your back will never make you wrong. They are there to support you in your choice regardless of what it is.

A person that makes you wrong for a choice, while saying they have your back, is not kind. They are judgmental. They are saying that they only have your back if you make a choice that they agree with. I'm sorry, that is scoundrel. Many people pretend to have your back and as soon as the situation gets a place that makes them uncomfortable, they make you wrong or create trauma and drama. You might find them saying, "I told you so", "You never listen to me" or "I told you he was a bad person." You don't need people like that in your life. They are not people that have your back; they are just people that take up space in your life and don't really contribute in any way.

I met someone recently whom everyone was calling a very kind gentleman. On looking at how he was acting and the things that he was saying, he was so out of touch as to what was actually going on. He was so vested in saying the right things at the right time and *always* giving the other person choice that he allowed his life to be continually swayed by the choices of others. Where was he in the picture? He actually wasn't there at all. Kindness, from his point of view, was where he did everything that the other person asked and when he was presented with a choice, he would refuse to make a choice. There was no kindness for him. He had no sense of what he actually required. He only delivered what others required. When a person does this, they have no sense of self. They have no way of creating a life without someone else giving all the directions. His partner is getting frustrated because he's not stepping up and being the man that she desires. She desires for him to make a choice for him but his continual refusal is creating friction in the relationship. She was commenting to me that he is at the beck and call of his mother. Ah, so that's where it started. His mother has made him totally subservient to her and, thus, he has no choice but to do whatever she wishes. Is the mother kind? No, she is definitely not. She has created a son that has no sense of self. That is not kind, that again is scoundrel.

In this discussion about kindness, I have explored the meaning of kindness, the things people do to create kindness and the pretence of kindness. As I finish this off, let me leave you with a few questions that will allow you to begin to create a life that is kind and free of abuse.

Am I being kind to me?

When you ask this question, it allows you to being to see whether you are actually being kind to you. Is it a kindness to you to stay in a relationship that doesn't work? No. Is it a kindness to you to stay in a job that you don't like? No. Is it a kindness to you to have some time by yourself reflecting the way your life is going? Yes. When you ask this question, you start to become aware of where there is kindness in your life and where there is not.

When you are with a person, you can ask:

Is this kind or operating from the pretense of kindness?

If after asking the question, you become aware of whether the person is actually kind or acting with the pretense of kindness. If the person has the pretense of kindness, you then have choice as to stay or go as you please. If you find that the person is operating under a pretense, please do not confront them with it.

They may not even be aware of it themselves. And, if you do, you may have a confrontation on your hands. The awareness is just for you. When you ask such a question, you have choice as to stay or go as you choose.

Unkindness is also a choice. Kindness is a choice. Any person can choose to be unkind or kind as they choose. What will you choose? Will you choose to be kind to you?

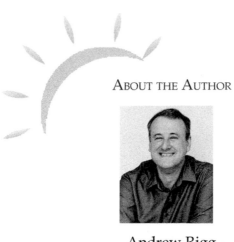

About the Author

Andrew Rigg

Andrew Rigg is a Leader, Project Creator, Facilitator, Radio Show Host and Gentleman inviting new possibilities to people across the world. He loves facilitating people to new and exciting possibilities, whether individually or in a group. His target is to create a world where abuse no longer exists and where kindness, gratitude and joy are predominant energies.

Offering private sessions, Andrew assists you to dissolve and release limiting beliefs and blocks that hold you back from creating and generating with ease the life you want to experience.

Drawing mainly upon Access Consciousness® tools and processes, but also incorporating Access Bars® Sessions, Access Consciousness® Body Processes, Symphony of Possibilities and Access Consciousness classes.

Andrew is an Access Consciousness® Certified Facilitator, Access Consciousness® Body Process Facilitator, Right Body For You Taster Facilitator and Founder of Happy Humanoids Radio.

After an extended illness in the late 1990s where doctors, therapists and healers couldn't identify what was happening, Andrew enrolled himself into a Reiki course not having any idea of what Reiki was about. Overnight, the illness changed. Andrew pursued many different energy healing techniques, developed a few energy healing techniques of his own and then came to Access Consciousness®.

Andrew was a public servant for almost 20 years in the both the Australian Capital Territory Government and Australian Government where he held many different roles. He was always looking for something that he actually liked doing.

* Access Consciousness® Certified Facilitator
* Access Consciousness® Body Process Facilitator
* Creator of Happy Humanoid Radio show
* Creator of Gentleman, Relationships, Choice Radio show
* Bachelor of Applied Science (chemistry major)
* Developed various energy healing techniques, especially Unity Templates and Nature Spirit Healing
* Reiki Master
* Shamballa Multi-dimensional Healing Master
* Practitioner of Melchizedek Method, Gaiadon Heart, Golden Triangle Healing, Isis Blue Moon Healing, Drisana™, Archangel activations and many other energy techniques
* EFT & TFT practitioner
* Polarity Therapist
* Former Kinesiologist having practiced and studied Touch For Health IV, Kinergetics Level 7, SFEF Kinesiology, Applied Physiology and Counselling Kinesiology
* Married to Eri Rigg, a most wonderful lady
* Father of Braden
* Stepfather to Hayley, Mari and Yuka

You can learn more about Andrew at:
http://www.accessrigg.com.au/
http://www.andrewrigg.space/

Please contact Andrew at:
andrew@accessrigg.com.au

CHAPTER 9

Relinquishing My Crown

Betsy McLoughlin

You are beautiful. Yes, YOU! You are kind, generous, brilliant, funny and lovable. You are amazing JUST as you are. If you are asking how could I possibly know this since I've never met you – I KNOW – I just do! It's an awareness that we all have these things within us. You might have hidden these traits until it was safe to bring them back - YOU are all these things and much more.

I longed to hear those words as a child. I desired to hear that I could do anything I wanted to – that I was strong, capable, and beautiful inside and out. I longed for my mother to enfold me in her arms in deep, loving hugs that never happened. I waited for the day she would tell me she loved me no matter what size my body was – I bet you can guess I never heard those words. It didn't occur to me then that I could tell myself all the things I looked for others to tell me-- that I could hug myself and nurture ME with all the love I had inside, no matter what my circumstances were in the moment.

For a long time I ran away from the words "abuse survivor". I didn't want to admit that I had been abused. The truth is I had experienced many forms of abuse in my life – physical, emotional, verbal, and sexual. I also heaped a bunch of self-abuse to ensure I stayed permeated in the muck. I added it like whipped cream and a cherry on top of the ice cream sundae. I felt such shame around this that I did my best to pretend that none of the abuse happened. I wanted to be "normal" without my perceived stigma of that label.

The picture painted by my adopted parents of our life was that of a happy, middle class family with three children, a dog, cats and a white picket fence. In reality, life was the opposite. Control, anger, hatred and alcoholism ruled the day. I assumed my role as the oldest sibling was to show my brother and sister how to pretend that all was good. I did my best to shelter them from the short fuses of both parents and allow them as normal a life as possible in the toxic environment we called home. I walked on eggshells never knowing what might possibly tip the scales so I wouldn't be on the receiving end of whatever violence or horrible words might be directed at me. I felt it was my duty to endure the brunt of the abuse since I was the oldest and I could handle it.

I became an amazing actress – putting on the appearance that I had no cares in the world – the "happy go lucky" girl. I pretended that life at home was wonderful. I fragmented myself to the different parts of my life – school, boyfriend, work and home. No one knew about the abuse – not even my boyfriend. There was an unspoken rule that we never discussed the abuse or alcoholism - not even at home. For a brief period in high school, Dad went to Alcoholics Anonymous. As usual, this was hidden from us – I only discovered this by accident – I came across an AA manual stashed away in a bookcase. I was so confused as to why they would keep this secret. Isn't going to AA a good thing? A step in the right direction?

Shame ran rampant in the household and I adopted the attitude of shame also. What if I was simply aware of my parent's shame? Now I know that I had nothing to be ashamed of.

Did you buy the point of view that you were wrong growing up as I did? Did you believe that you could never do anything right? Did you always feel that you had a heavy cloud of abuse hovering over you?

Conclusions...

I was given up for adoption when I was a few days old. I received my birth mother's intake papers from the California Children's Home when I was an adult. These papers revealed the tiniest glimmer of my mother. She chose not to tell anyone about my existence, including my birth father. The papers also showed she developed toxemia during her pregnancy with me. When I read this, I began sobbing and felt connected to her for the first time EVER.

I cried because when I was pregnant I also developed toxemia and was on bed rest for the last two months of my pregnancy. Toxemia occurs when your blood pressure goes dangerously high; it can be life threatening for both mother and child. I had no records of any family health problems and always wondered if my birth mother had any similar pregnancy issues. This tiny connection with her and the ensuing tears surprised me. They felt cathartic and I let them fall as I felt an unknown wall disappear.

After being adopted by a wealthy family (I will call them family #2), I was only with them for a couple of months before the head of the household discovered he had a terminal illness, at which point they decided they could not raise me. Family #2 took me back to the Children's Home where a foster mother (family #3) cared for me until the couple who became my "permanent" parents (family #4) adopted me when I was six months old. Just a little confusing for a child to wrap her head around. Am I confusing you telling the story? Haha!

Having heard this story as a child, I decided that I was unlovable and that no one wanted me; everyone abandoned me and always would. This one conclusion was the basis for a great amount of turmoil and angst in my life. How do you NOT have any type of relationship with the person who gave birth to you?

I decided being adopted was strange in the sense that I had no reference points. I had no idea who my grandparents were, if I had aunts and uncles or siblings. Who was my father? What did they look like? What were their personalities like? I made that significant and I concluded that I was floating around like a balloon without a string with no family ties. I excluded my adoptive family #4 from the family ties.

Have you ever noticed that when you conclude something, it closes the door to other options? You've walked away from that door when possibly there were other doors you could choose.

Queen of Victimland

I crowned myself Queen of Victimland. I spent most of my life in this role and I wore my crown proudly. With justifications for all the choices I made, I kept myself Queen by perpetuating all of my conclusions and judgments of how awful my life had been. I felt sorry for myself.

After all, I rationalized - who has four families before six months of age? Who gets adopted into a family that has alcohol abuse, verbal, physical and sexual abuse? Looking at everything from this point of view perpetuated the thoughts that I must be an awful person! I definitely deserved this since I was so unlovable.

Toxic environments necessitate special adaptive skills. You teach yourself how to negotiate the bumpy roads of never knowing what you are going to encounter when you walk through the front door. You learn to be hyper sensitive to the moods of everyone in the house. You become the peacekeeper and learn to neglect your own needs, burying any desires you might have. Anticipating needs were also a must. ANYTHING to ensure you weren't going to be the recipient of a beating or hours of verbal abuse OR both. Keep them calm. Keep them happy – no matter what! Many times I was so confused about why I was being punished - I had absolutely nothing to do with whatever angered them and I was an easy target.

I concluded that I must be a horrible person to be in this family. I must deserve all the anger and vitriol directed at me. *I'll be better next time. I won't make you angry, I'm sorry. Please don't hit me. Please stop drinking. Please stop yelling. I can't take this.*

Time for Change

This is a snapshot of my life growing up and the choices I made. I have changed my life completely. I am no longer afraid that I will make mistakes – I embrace them and laugh at how serious I could become over miniscule events. What if life could be joyous? As I began asking that question, different possibilities emerged.

How did I go from tiptoeing around the outskirts of my life to living a life full of joy? The first thing I did was GLADLY relinquish my crown of Queen of that lonely and remote land of Victimland. I burned down the fortress of walls erected. I chose to live my life and no longer be an observer from the outside looking in.

I disengaged from the toxic relationships I had built when I thought I couldn't do any better. That included ending some friendships and a marriage. I asked lots of questions about whether that person was a contribution to me and vice versa. I have also reinvented my definition of friendship for something that worked for me. I am no longer the whipping post for anyone's frustrations, I have removed the doormat from my back.

Now I ask for generative and creative relationships. And... the people who have shown up in my life have been beyond any expectations. I truly feel blessed and grateful.

I STOPPED doubting my awareness, my intuition, and my gut instinct. It has never let me down. I used to pooh pooh this intuition and invariably whenever I did, things would go haywire. Now even if it doesn't make sense, I listen to the whispers of intuition or knowing.

When I chose to change my life, miracles have unfolded in all kinds of yummy ways. I chose to STOP all forms of abuse in my life – even the ones I used to think were "little" or "minor" that I allowed. I chose to END the cycle of abuse with my son. Who knows how many generations of abuse I came from – that we all come from! I remember clearly as a teenager saying quite firmly – I will NOT physically or sexually abuse my children or allow this to continue – and I haven't.

I ended my self-abuse and I said NO to any more self-loathing behavior. I looked at myself as never before. I saw the beautiful, generous, kind, sweet, fun and loving person I truly am – as we all are.

I stopped making myself wrong for everything. If I find myself slipping into old patterns, I ask "what else can you choose here?" and I don't berate me for anything that I've done. It's all a choice. What if there is no judgable offense? What freedom!

A question that occurred to me was "What if you are so much stronger than you ever gave yourself credit for?" This question changed so much for me. For the first time, I began to look at that possibility, to realize how strong I truly was. From this strength, I began to choose for me and not against me.

I began a search for self-discovery and found Reiki. This modality was wonderful and I jumped in to learning all I could and became a Reiki Master. Continuing the quest for more, I found Access Consciousness®. Here is what I had been looking for – learning how to empower ME without expectations.

Access offers many amazing tools for your life including body processes and Access Bars®. This process is a gentle hands-on process for 32 points on your head. This process changed my life. For the first time since I could remember, the chatter of my "monkey mind" was quiet. My body felt nurtured, adored and my life truly became so much more than I ever thought was possible. I no longer felt depressed and suicidal thoughts quickly went away and have never returned! How amazing is that?

I had NO idea this was possible with such ease. It was so different than all the years of therapy and medications I had tried. I had been to a couple therapists and they were quick to prescribe anti-depressants. For me, medications numbed me and made me feel more disconnected and was exactly the opposite of what I was looking for. I discontinued medications and continued my quest for myself and joy that I knew I would uncover. I did find an amazing therapist who contributed so much to me for a couple years.

I was quite fortunate to find some amazing facilitators that assisted me as I continued healing. Layers of doubt and hatred peeled away and my beauty unfolded in front of me like a beautiful rose. All the things I had hidden away surfaced with joy. I faced the sun with the delicious warmth on my skin - so grateful I had chosen to stay in this beautiful world.

Now I nurture and adore me. I embrace ALL sides of me. I giggle when I find myself controlling something and ask one of my favorite questions "What else is possible here?"

Questions invite possibilities and awareness and for me, that is empowering! Here are some questions for you to consider – don't look for an answer. Questions are designed to get you out of thinking and into playing with the multitude of possibilities.

What would your life look like if you didn't change you for anyone?

What if you don't shut yourself off to please others?

What if you don't have to do anything you don't want to do?

What would your life look like if you stayed true to YOU – no matter what?

What are you good at that you've never considered?

What brings you joy?

What contribution are you to your friends, family and work?

Would you be willing to be kind to you?

Would you be willing to be grateful for you?

Would you be willing to be grateful for all your choices that have led you to where you are now?

I invite you to consider different possibilities around the energy of abuse. No longer do you have to twist yourself inside out like a pretzel to fit to the requirements of everyone else in your life.

I am truly grateful that I chose beyond the label of abuse – that I chose beyond my past into an exciting present and future! My past does not define me any longer. I share the story so you know you can overcome whatever it is in your life that may have stopped you.

What else is truly possible my beautiful, sweet, powerful friend? What else?

About the Author

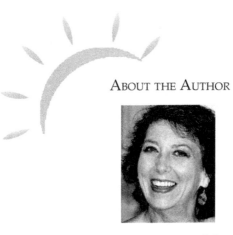

Betsy McLoughlin

Betsy McLoughlin is a #1 international best-selling author (this marks Betsy's sixth book), a radio show host and an Access Consciousness® Certified Facilitator. She is a Transformational Coach, a Body Process Facilitator®, Right Body for You® Taster Facilitator and so much more! Her vibrant personality is the space of no judgment and is the catalyst for quicker success and happiness for her clients.

This creator of magnitude has been featured on The *Ask BonBon TV Show*, numerous radio shows and tele-summits. The radio show Betsy co-hosts, *Imperfect Brilliance*, can be found on YouTube.

Betsy is also a magical Realtor® who creates ease for her clients. Her calm demeanor, willingness to ask questions outside the box and look for what else is possible creates more opportunities for her clients.

Betsy would love to create new possibilities with you. Are you ready? You can email her at accessbetsy@gmail.com. Check out her websites at www.creatingyumminess.com and www.imperfectbrilliance.com.

CHAPTER 10

Set the World on Fire

Melanie Meade

Sunrise, I awake. I open my eyes to the dazzling brightness, the beauty and the clarity my eyes are not used to seeing. It has been a while. I shade my eyes from the intensity as if I had just come out of my cocoon and adjust to my surroundings and what I now see. My restful slumber is done. I am recharged, refreshed and inspired and I see the possibilities in what is the beginning of a beautiful life. I stretch out my arms and greet the dawn. A long awaited welcome, like long lost friends reunited. I inhale the deep, fresh dewy air that boosts my sleepy body. It injects a joy, that zest for life and I am once again enthusiastic, anticipating the adventures that await.

The intense, still silence of the dawn is a haunting reminder of my now quiet mind. A world of peace and ease that I had evaded for so long, no longer filled with the noise of shoulds and judgments and the chaos of this reality. I now get to choose and I choose to fill it with the beauty the simplicity of life, like the dawn chorus as birds sing in solo and in unison, the gentle, refreshing breeze which re-energises me and washes me clean of what is not mine. It gifts me a sense of peace that is missed by the weary as they sleep on. How did I get so lucky to wake up to such beauty and peace around me and now also within? The world does not look the same as it used to.

As I continue to awaken the sun gently continues to rise, glowing and greeting me, inviting me to more of life, more of me and more of what I know. For the sun will shine no matter what, whether you bask in it or seek shade it blazes bright regardless and invites you more to live. It has a certain magnetism to it that I adore.

I gratefully greet the world, feeling more alive now and wonder what grand and glorious adventures await.

For this is just the beginning… a fresh start for a fuller life, more of me, more of what I once knew was possible.

I was once, and maybe still at times, too much and rather than blaze brightly I chose to quench my flame. Though the embers always smouldered, I ignored it. I never tended to it. I never stoked them or dare even acknowledge their existence or contemplate re-igniting them.

I buried that fire, that brightness in the depths of my being. Rather than set the world on fire I ached and the bright promises of possibilities were written into fairy tale. It was a dark secret only kept to myself, never to be revealed. A sleeping beauty that lay in repose, such a beauty that was so natural to me yet terrified others.

The truth is you cannot hide that which is truly you no matter how hard you try. I would intrigue people and once they captured the essence of my true beauty they recoiled, repulsed and reacted just like the villain in the fairy tales I read as a child. Banished to the outer reaches of this reality, and I with it. Rather than receive and bask in the warmth and kindness they were scorched by the intensity, it agonised people. It would swiftly change from fascination at something they have never seen before to a repulsion, at times requiring very dramatic action and I would stand there confused by the commotion, never fully grasping what I was creating for others. I meant to harm.

This beauty inside me started feeling like a curse I carried with me as it only seemed to create pain and this saddened me that is what it created. It had to be me that was creating this and I no longer wished to inflict this pain in the world. I was the common denominator.

This was a world that made no sense to me. My joy became a secret and gradually those bursts of dazzling fireworks turned to a fizzle and eventually I felt nothing. The choice to stop and to quench that exuberance created a lot of pain and anxiety for me. That flame that blazed so naturally, that danced and flickered with the joy of living, that exuded warmth and welcome, that had a beauty and innocence to it was doused by this reality.

What I found the most challenging was no matter how hard I tried to hide it, a spark of brilliance remained. I could not see it anymore, I did not want to but an essence of it lingered, it could not be completely quashed or quelled. It intrigued others and would draw them toward me with curious eyes and an uncomfortable level of fascination with me.

They would look and seek and search and with loving words, offers of friendship, affections and promises of futures. Without warning all that would change instead it would get twisted into something else. From outright rejection and ridicule to other more intense anger it would leave me in a spin. Some from people I knew and some from complete strangers. I never felt entirely safe.

I had been threatened to be killed, harmed, destroyed, segregated, divided and separated. They tried to control, subdue, dumb me down, make me worthless and told I was nothing but an embarrassment and would never amount to anything. I could recant stories of years of bullying, of humiliation, of public attacks, berated and jeered at in front of peers, of isolation and separation and so forth. The end result was the searing anguish of existence in a world that felt I could not burn bright in as I would burn and be destroyed.

How do you not be you? Amidst the confusion I withdrew and closed off. I shut down. I waited – for exactly what I could not say other than this world was not for me nor I for it. I felt small and hopeless and I believed everything I had been told for I no longer could not see another way. I was lost in this reality rapidly losing confidence of a way out and of a life I knew was possible, once upon a time.

Who was I? What was I doing? Was this really it? Was everyone else right? Life seemed to be happening to me, it was out of my control, I could not reign it in and change it. A tsunami of wrongness and doubt enveloped my world leaving me merciless to where ever life pulled me. I did not know what to grab onto, what could I do to save myself from drowning?

It was not just one life altering event, it was a cycle of wrongness I ended up in that opened the door to years of great unhappiness as others felt it necessary to inflict their pain onto me for me to burden and carry. It became one thing after another and a complete blur. I could not tell you which and what and when as it became normal.

From a young age it became one soul destroying experience after another, all varying in degrees of intensity but enough to shatter my spirit and keep me locked up in my cycle of wrongness and helplessness with a feeling of no way out. I would attempt to go quietly about my life but I could not avoid the land mines. It was like no matter where I turned I would step on one and detonate it. I lived in a state of hyper vigilance and isolation and chose the devil I knew rather than the devil I didn't.

They seemed like my only choices at the time and I chose the lesser of two evils or so I hoped.

I was sensitive. I was bright. I had an optimism about me. I saw the world my way. This was not appealing to others and I eventually lost my optimism, it was not fun for me anymore. I had to hide my way of being and it felt safer to conform and that in itself was a disaster. I was terrible at it. I quietened down, I tried to hide, I withdrew. I found people difficult, so friendships were not easy for me as they took their own course too and I preferred to minimise those experiences. Needless to say that made school an unpleasant experience. I was bullied for years, by both students and teacher. Even when I changed schools the damage had been done. That summer in between changing schools I spent those bright and sunny months locked away in my room. I did not want to go outside, see or even talk to people. This was the only way I could find peace and it wasn't going to be the last time I would resort to total isolation. I ached too much inside and it was all I knew how to make life easier on me. I felt so horrendous and out of place all I could do was try get through school. University didn't last long, just a year. I found living quite an ordeal. While everyone else was out spreading their wings with life experiences I struggled. This world was not at all I thought it to be as a child. It was like I was sold a lie, which I bought hook, line and sinker.

One wonderful, beautiful gift came into my life, my son. Being his mother gave me a sense of hope. I wanted the world for him. I wanted him to thrive no matter what – everywhere I had failed was still a possibility for him. He just brightened my world. No one was going to stop him being him.

When he was 1 I had a car accident. This was to slam the brakes on any little bit of momentum in my life. I had done enough damage to myself and the car to have sustained injuries whereby my body could barely move. It hurt so bad. Talking, thinking, walking and everyday functioning ached. My son brought me solace, he kept me going. That desire for him had not faded and no amount of pain was going to stop me from being a mother to him. No one or nothing would ever interfere with that and in a life of what felt like helplessness there lay my seed of strength, that desire for something greater. I could get out of bed for him and go about my day for him. I did not want him to suffer for it. I kept going.

He was all I loved about my life. What I was then living is not how I wanted to live, it all kind of just happened. I did not like the necessity of having to shut down and shut off to life, it felt my safest option my whole life and there I was after doing my best to not cause attract drama and it was occurring anyway. People seemed to capitalise on my sickness it almost put fire in their belly to up the ante on me, kick me while I was down.

When I was being me it created commotion and when I would stop it created a lot of unhappiness for me and the commotion continued. I was surrounded by mean, uncaring, narcissistic people and all that seemed greater than what beauty was in my life. Maybe I felt I didn't deserve the morsel of that for myself.

I was constantly tormented by other people taking out their own issues on me. I did not want the life I was living. It wasn't working for me, I knew there was something else available. This lifestyle I fell into was all chosen by necessity. I was squashed into the tiniest box but the alternative to break free seemed too traumatic. My body was slow, I had enough strength to go about my day and make sure my son had the best possible life available to him. My money was disappearing, my bills spiralled to the point I could no longer afford the physiotherapy treatment I had been getting for those few years that my body required. The physical agony matched my agony of existence. It was like a distraction from my unhappiness it was so painful my main thoughts were to just get through the day. I grew more isolated, I could not cope with the anxiety of going outside unless I had to. I was just about functioning and I was screaming inside for something different and so was my body. I just didn't know how.

When this is what the world is how do I live my own reality, the one I knew was possible as a small child?

I awoke one morning, amidst all this intensity and opened my eyes and realised for the first time in years there was no pain. For those moments there was no mental anguish. I could just get out of bed, I could just walk down the stairs, I could run and play with my little boy and enjoy every movement free from the mind numbing restriction I had for years. I finally got a sense of what was possible for me. I remember those sensations from when I was young. When the sun blazed bright and warmed my skin, I would smile and look up at the sky and feel free. I would run and play without a care in the world as it was my world and nothing else mattered, I was me!

From that moment on I started choosing different. My body was far from healed. That morning was a short lived glimpse of what was possible but enough to remind me of my dreams, what I once knew was true. I did not take drastic or abrupt action. But what I did start doing was taking baby steps in caring for myself more. The drama continued around me and I grew increasingly weary of it. I could not figure out why it was going on, it was like it was drawn toward me but I kept choosing towards that sense of freedom and joy I sensed that morning I woke and my world, though briefly, was different. I welcomed me back into the world again – step by step, back to living my life.

I took my time, choosing for me again and almost anticipating those reactions that occurred when I chose to shut myself down when I was young. It was tentative. It wasn't easy and still sometimes it isn't.

No matter what we choose, whether it is to stay or go or maybe wait a little longer – whatever it is that is going on for you – no one is greater than you. No one and nothing has power over you – it is you who gets to choose how to be with situations – and none of it is wrong. We do the best we know how at that time.

I chose towards that sense of peace and strength I knew I had, somewhere. I just kept going, even when I felt terrible, even when I felt worthless, even when I felt wrong.

Being you can be scary, as it is something we can refuse and suppress. It can be terrifying for others when we truly be – as it is something the world has never seen before. It challenges others to stretch out of their comfort zones and be their own greatness too. It's a new experience. There is no handbook for what's to come. But what if you couldn't fail?

Choosing for you and toward the life you desire to create does not promise those pats on the back, the reassurances of how great you are, that you are doing well and on the right path. Please do not seek them and keep going.

It has not rid my life of pains or problems but I do get to choose how I be with them and they are minor irritations in my life now. There are people who are willing me on in life to be more, go farther and explore what else is possible for me. Though few, they are a gift I am truly grateful for.

Life ebbs and flows, it chops and changes often with no warning. There is no final destination so please do not look where you need to be and ride that wave – just choose and keep on going. Keep putting one foot in front of the other whether you are crawling, walking or running.

I awoke that morning and I felt like the beginning of something new. I took my time and trusted me. Sometimes I dragged myself through but something greater would always show up. The only way I know is forward, no matter what.

My days are filled with the possibility of peace that long eluded me, of a joy I once knew existed and a life I am choosing towards to burn brightly!

I cannot tell you how to create that other than the sun does not apologise for shining, even if it blinds you. Be that! People will choose how to be with that, you do not get to control that outcome. They will adjust to their liking and the sun just keeps burning effortlessly. Some will shade themselves from you and other will enjoy your flame, your warmth, your radiance and will encourage you to shine even brighter. No matter what you just keep shining. For you being you is the greatest gift to you and to others. It is what will truly change this world. You cannot cause harm by being brilliant, being bright and being the beauty that you are.

Nothing is real. Nothing is fixed or solid. Nothing is greater than your choice. You are not tied to anything nor is there one way to go about creating your beautiful life.

"Go forth and set the world on fire" – Rumi

Burn bright. Burn brilliant.

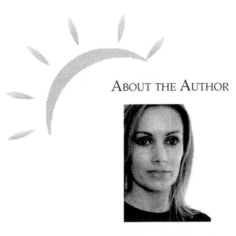

ABOUT THE AUTHOR

Melanie Meade

Realising an ordinary life was not always going to work for her, Melanie is on a journey of what else is truly possible. She is a rule breaker but not in the conventional sense of the word. Never good at the order of life Melanie breaks the boundaries as an out of the box thinker.

Her journey has taken her from a local government law office into the arena of personal development and international communications and marketing roles working alongside like-minded and inspiring game changers who are spreading their message worldwide. Melanie is also a #1 bestselling author sharing her unique perspective on how she sees the world.

Melanie invites you to a life where you have the simplicity and gentleness that change can be. Where the ease of creating is second-nature and where you get to be the magic of you, whether anyone sees it or not. What if your life could be bigger that you've ever imagined?

melaniemeade.com

CHAPTER 11

Changing DNA

Wendy Terry

The moment I laid eyes on him again everything changed, I changed. In that moment it felt like I had been hit by a lightning bolt – I felt my whole being change right down to my DNA. How could this be happening? I had just been reunited with my first love after 32 years.

I looked at him and from deep within my soul I knew I had to be with him. My love for him was so deep; like nothing I had ever felt before – but how could this be? I was happily married - I had been married for over 27 years. I had a life in Canada with my husband and our 3 beautiful girls. I had returned to my roots in England for a holiday; I was shaken to my core!

In the moment that I laid eyes on this man I could easily have had sex with him, right then and right there; this was something that was so out of character for me. I had never had a one night stand before and chose to only have sex when I was in a committed relationship. I had never had sex with this man. I had been too young – or had I been? Because during the 19 months that we went out together I had been raped at the tender age of 14 – something I kept from him and everyone else. My virginity had been stolen from the person I loved the most.

Upon my return to Canada I became sad. I knew I was dying inside. I was not the same person anymore. I longed to be with this man. I tried so hard to fight it. I was being ripped apart inside. Torn in two – I had a love for my family and a love for this man.

This man himself had just gotten out of a 20-year marriage; a marriage where his wife chose to have an affair and get pregnant with her lover's child and then moved her lover in with her, her husband and their child. This man tried to get out but his lawyer told him he had to remain where he was so he could get some equity out of the house. After four months he could no longer take it. When he heard his wife making love in the next bedroom with her lover it was like a knife cutting through him. This was all too much to handle; his wife would abuse him emotionally and physically. He in turn allowed this, as he would never hit back to anyone, let alone a pregnant woman. He finally left, scared and depleted but ready to start anew.

After six months his wife asked him to go back, she told him she still loved him – even though she was still living with the father of her new baby. This man chose to take some of his power back and for the first time said NO!

This man knew what a broken marriage felt like so he did not want to break up a marriage but all he knew was he wanted to be with me – it was so deep in is soul. The night he reconnected with me he went home and cried, well actually he did not cry he sobbed; something he had not done before – he was shaken to his core!

We started to write letters to each other which progressed into phone calls. I was amazed at how well he seemed to know me even though I was only 13 and he was 15 when we started dating all those years ago. We talked and talked and could not stop. We had so much to catch up on. I found the courage to tell him about my rape; his response made me cry as he was so concerned and asked if anyone was there for me at the time. He was the only one who had ever said that to me. At the time of the rape I thought it was my fault, I had let someone buy me a drink while I was away on holiday with family and a friend. Looking back on it later in life I realized the male must have put something in my drink; it was not my fault at all. I was so naive in my younger years, trusting and believing everyone. Why would anyone want to do something "bad" to someone else? By telling my first love about my rape it helped me heal that piece from deep within. I felt my first love knew me inside out, better than anyone else on this earth. I could not get this man out of my mind; it was like he had possessed my mind and my soul!

I went on holiday by myself to England so I could see him. My husband was understanding and allowed this he told me to get it out of my system. I went and it just confirmed what I knew in the moment I connected to this man – I loved him.

I returned to Canada again and felt even sadder inside. I was pretending to everyone. People would say to me; you look fantastic, you are beaming, you have such a glow. I thought if only you knew why – something had opened up deep inside of me – I was deeply in love!

I would look at my family knowing the truth – that I wanted to go back to England and be with this man but how could I leave them?

I started to abuse me with my thinking. I began tearing myself apart – I hated me for doing this to my family. They were kind and loving and deserved so much more. I felt like a bad person and a bad mother. Two of my daughters had left home and were living with their boyfriends but I still had a 17-year-old at home.

I could not stand the torture, inside I felt like I was dying.

Being a psychic medium I have great knowing – I knew if I stayed I would get cancer and physically die. I knew if I went I would metaphorically die but I would renew. My family would at least physically have me here.

I told my husband I wanted to go to England to be with this man. He told me to go; he would wait six months for me. I told him no – I would be going to have sex with another man and he should respect himself more. Even if it did not work out with me and this man I chose this man over him and he should not settle.

Some of my family were so upset with me, they swore at me and shouted at me and one even hit me. I allowed it as I understood their pain. I understood how shocked they were as I was just as shocked this happened to me. I understood how scared they were.

I left with emotions coming up in every direction; happy, sad, nervous, excited and so much more.

Just before I left, my friend taught me about emotional releasing, including how to release sadness. We were out for a drive and stopped along a river. We sat down to do some releasing and lot of dragonflies swarmed up around us - it was magical.

I continued to release the sadness every day. I cried and I cried, I sobbed and I sobbed. I had never cried from the well of my soul before. On some level I was the happiest I had ever been while on another level the saddest because I was away from my daughters.

I returned to Canada after 6 months. My husband had a girlfriend by this time and I was happy that we were amicable. My girlfriend worked with him on emotional releasing so he was able to move on. I stayed in the spare room of our marital home where my husband and daughter lived. I let my husband stay there for the sake of our daughter as I did not want to disrupt her any more than necessary. I knew she was hurting. I would go into her bedroom and I could feel all her pain and heartache. I would cry wondering why did this have to happen to her. Why did I have to do this to my family? I would shout at my angels, guides and loved ones "you better make sure my girls are ok or else I can't do this!" I knew somewhere there was a higher purpose even though I did not understand it all at the time.

I returned to England and continued to release my emotions. I got to the deeper ones; emotions I never knew existed, emotions I was unaware of. I kept going deeper and deeper – being very truthful with myself and my feelings.

One day I felt very alone; even though I had a man who loved me and our relationship was the easiest and happiest I had ever been in; he was at work and I had to go through my emotions alone. I went to the park where a young girl had come to swing on the swing beside me; she was very sweet and reminded me of one of my daughters at her age. This bought up so many memories and I went home and sobbed. It was painful – I wanted to die. I understood why people would choose suicide – and then in that instant when I felt like I could take no more I felt myself break open. I felt the pure essence of me emerge – I was free!

I stopped feeling bad. I was and had always been a good mother. I loved my children unconditionally. I went back to Canada twice a year to see them. I could still be there for them if they chose so.

My relationship with my first love is so happy and easy. I al-

ways thought a good relationship meant you had to compromise; in our relationship there is no compromise as we are always on the same page. We really do love the same things and
have the same taste. When picking out anything for our condo
we always choose the same things. We both love simplicity. We
have the kind of relationship where one could finish one's sentence for the other one or if I want him to pick up something on
the way home I only have to think it and he often does it. We
are silly and fun. We did not have a lot of spare money when
we first got together so we created ways to have fun without
spending very much. We love picnics indoors and outdoors
along with water pistol fights. We play snakes and ladders with
a twist amongst other games. We have told each other "I love
you" in hundreds of ways. We are very romantic towards each
other in ways that cost little or nothing. We love talking and
listening to each other, both respecting each other's points of
view, going for walks and our favourite past time of all; going
to the beach and watching the waves – something to do on any
day. We allow each other to just be. We have always compli-
mented each other on our strengths; we get along so well and
never really argue. This is the easiest relationship we have ever
been in. We bring the best out in each other and appreciate every single moment together. I love how the energy just flows
between us, lifting each other to new heights.

From this process I chose more of me; I chose to look deep inside of me; I chose to release my core emotions so they could be
freed from my cell memory, from my DNA. I chose to see the
good the bad and the ugly inside of me. By doing this I was able
to see all aspects of other people and free their energy blocks. I
could see with clients that some were past life issues, while
some had ancestor issues that were carried energetically
through them. We all have emotional issues. Some people are
just unaware or choose not to look inside themselves – not
ready for the adventure that would lie ahead – not ready to go

to HAPPIER! I have released many issues in clients and many energy blocks. I was once told you can't change the past – you can't change what happened. It is up to you what you believe but I have taken clients through the glass of time so they can re-write their past. They can change anything about it; they have free will and control. What this does is change their energy from their cell memory. It releases the negative, heavy energy and clears it to lighter, healthier happier cells. It goes all the way down to the DNA –when it changes the DNA I see the strands change colour and straighten out.

So I don't believe that your energy, your DNA can't change. My DNA changed and yours can too!

I went from being happy to unlocking all my locked up emotions, some which had been hidden for years even centuries to being HAPPIER!

My life is so much easier now. I released drama which only complicates life. I let go of material things which causes a lot of stress for many people; and in the end does not matter. I chose not to take things personally as those emotions just get attached to you. If an emotion comes up, I look at me as it is never to do with anyone else they are just triggering that emotion in you. I am always grateful for that person who triggered the emotion that needed to be released. This always sends me to a higher, happier place. My heart fills with gratitude and love.

I know that if I had not chosen to do this journey I would never have looked so deeply inside of me, healing myself on many levels. This journey has shown that I can adapt to any circumstance. I have grown in leaps and bounds. I would never have stepped out of my comfort zone and even wrote this chapter. I would never have gone beyond what I thought was possible.

I am proud of myself and my family for doing this journey as it has taken great inner strength.

For those of us choosing to really learn our souls will evolve so we can go to a different higher happier level when we die. I know because I have seen this. Look out for my upcoming book "The different levels of death and suicide" where I go into more detail about true life experiences and what I have seen.

I am free, may you find your freedom also.

ABOUT THE AUTHOR

About the Author

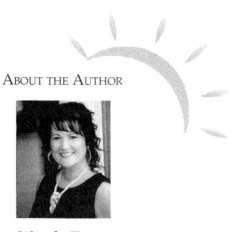

Wendy Terry

I was born in Cornwall, England, and lived in Bodmin. From a very young age, I have always seen spirits. "Why can I see faces and people when no one else in my family can?" I asked myself. What exactly was wrong with me? I would ask my friends if they saw colours or faces before them and the answer was always no. Soon, I stopped asking.

Afraid of the Night

I hated sleeping alone, and was always terrified. Often waking up in the night, I would fake a stomach ache just so I could reach to my mum for comfort. Though I had two wonderful brothers, I desperately wished for a sister who could share my room and prevent me from feeling so scared and alone. I simply didn't understand, nor did anyone in my family – none of us knew anyone who had experienced the gift I possess.

Finding Answers

When I was about 12 years old, my family moved into a house next to a tea leaf reader. I would visit her and be fascinated when, taking my tea cup, she would reveal a number of things. How could she see so much from a simple bunch of tea leaves? I am extremely grateful to her for opening up an entirely new avenue in my life. I enjoyed her readings, and became fascinated by the world of mediumship.

A Whole New World

At the age of 15, I moved to Canada with my family. It was there that my world really began to expand and open up. I loved visiting readers, and deeply appreciated their open and communal atmosphere.

Discovering My Calling

After I had my children, I started to read tarot cards. Soon, the spirits began to attend my readings. I went to a meditation class, which exposed me to another new world of fascination. Learning and growing continuously, I eventually began teaching what I had learned.

Sharing My Knowledge

I am extraordinarily passionate about teaching people to feel better about themselves, and giving them a different perspective on things. Teaching clients to listen to themselves, I open them up to their own innate abilities. My life recently brought me back to England – meaning I now travel between two beautiful countries performing work that I love. I am incredible grateful for all of the experiences and people who have crossed my path to date as they have made me the person I am today.

wendy.terry444@hotmail.com
www.wendyterrypsychic.com

CHAPTER 12

Thriving Beyond Abuse when Surviving Isn't Enough

Heather Bell

I remember sitting on the front steps of our family home and it was almost dinnertime. We had just had the biggest argument in the 12 odd years we had been together, and it was on the front porch, as a public show, for all to see and hear. Previously I had spent most of my life hiding the years of abuse away from the world. I didn't like to argue, I didn't like the confrontation, the battle that always ensued. But this time, it was different. Everything was different and I was changing.

As I sat crying alone on the front steps trying to process what had just occurred, I thought this was the worst of it, screaming at each other but doing it away from the kids so they couldn't hear it. A few minutes later my husband stepped over me and asked what I wanted for dinner.

That was the point I felt the most worthless, like scum on the bottom of someone's shoe. The actual act of being stepped over in such a manner (not in the fun way you used to play at as kids when you were mucking about with your friends), eroded any value I saw in myself as a human being.

In that 10-second moment, that was the biggest catalyst for me to choose something different.

Growing up the youngest of five had its advantages. I spent a long time watching those around me choose for them and for others, sometimes the end result was what they had hoped it would be, sometimes it wasn't. I remember saying to people close to me that I was learning all the things that I didn't want. I had created a foundation for my life based on everything I was avoiding, and interestingly, what you are avoiding is invariably what you will create.

I was very good at creating abuse for myself. I was different, that was very evident from birth. At 10 pounds, 9 ounces and 23.5 inches long that was different by even those standards back then. I learnt very early if your growth is ahead then there's an expectation you are way more capable of doing things, regardless of your age. I was way more capable, capable of creating a life that challenged me, and my family, on multiple levels. Somehow, my capacity to cope in situations that are less than ideal was created at a very early age too. Even as little children we have the power of our choices and our creations, which is why it seems all the more difficult to swallow when it involves abuse.

I had a strong temperament as a child and often made it abundantly clear that I was demanding to be heard. In the 1970s the word autism was not bandied around very often. Whilst the disorder was known, it was still in its infancy in terms of really understanding what children with autism were about. It's no surprise it wasn't recognised that I am autistic. Too much sensory stimulation would drive me to lash out, to exhibit such poor behaviour that in those days smacking was a normal consequence. I used to hide the wooden spoon (pickle spoon in our house) in an attempt to delay it. It bought me some time but it also contributed to longer, harder punishment. Trying to convey to a busy family that my head never stopped, ever, was impossible. I would talk incessantly, inappropriately, laugh raucously at inappropriate things and moments, and was constantly reprimanded for being me. Once I started school I would constantly interrupt the class by answering out of turn and talking. I remember at one point adults would ask if I actually breathed. I never drew breath in trying to get my words out quickly, before someone would ask me to be quiet or shut up. By the time I was seven I had learnt that being quiet was what made people happy, and my attempts at being heard were dismissed.

Being a tomboy I was always playing in the street with the children in our neighbourhood, and I spent a great deal of time with other families. We were a close-knit neighbourhood. All the parents knew each other and all the kids, both young and old, would hang out at each other's houses. My siblings had a lot of after school activities and I would often stay at friends' houses to avoid having to tag along. That's when the sexual abuse started. It lasted 2-3 years, maybe more. I thought it was normal, I thought everyone did it. I was sworn to secrecy though, manipulated into believing I would be seen as the reason it had occurred and therefore no one would believe me even if I did tell. Staying silent was to be used by them as a weapon against me. I had created a life for myself where my voice was not considered a contribution - it was an annoyance. The further I withdraw from the conversation, the easier it became to be silent, and this was a lure. I had managed to lock everything away for safekeeping, to my own detriment.

I had a sweet tooth for lollies back then, still do, however it was a bargaining tool for the perpetrators. They gave me money to buy whatever I wanted at the local shops in exchange for silence. It was very effective. During this stage I started to steal money too, and stationery items from newsagents and department stores. I never really understood why I decided to steal stationery items, just one of those random things you do when you're easily influenced. Looking back it was just another avenue of escapism. The millions of thoughts racing through my head every moment of every day were dotted frequently with recurring images of the abuse. It was an outlet for me to not think about getting caught and having to talk about it. Part way through one of the perpetrators was caught in the act by my family. It was discussed and dealt with by the parents, or so they thought. This only aggravated the perpetrator who then decided to take his frustration out on me, through threats. It also made him far more cunning and manipulative.

As I matured through my teenage years it became clear to me that being myself was not a good choice. Every time I tried it, it backfired and the constant bullying at school and abuse at home continued. I loved my family but I didn't want to be part of it. Where would I go though? Who would want me around? Who would want to include me or spend time with me? I created an environment where regardless of who I was with it was easy to bully me. That was my normal. That was what I expected, that was what kept me going. I didn't know how to receive kindness and when someone tried, I would lash out and be mean and unkind. I perpetuated that which I had tried so hard to escape. At 17 I had endured my last beating with the wooden spoon and knew I couldn't continue to live with my family. My siblings had all left home and I was on my own now, and the drinking had increased and therefore so had the violence. It was then that I met someone eight years my senior and he was my ticket out... out of the frying pan and into the fire.

As much as I hated being manipulated by this man, I accepted it as normal. Every time I wanted to leave he manipulated me back in again. The emotional, psychological and financial abuse was like nothing I had ever experienced before. I was isolated and ostracized from everyone. I believed wholeheartedly that relationships were about committing 150 percent of you to make the other person happy. Cutting off all of me to keep the relationship alive was normal. In the early days of the relationship I thought exiting this reality was the best choice. When I tried, it simply created more abuse, and I was still alive. I was blamed for the sexual abuse, he felt I had deserved it and brought it on myself. By the time I was free of him, well living with him at least, I was a mess, and tried to take my life for a second time. It was at this time that I asked for help, professional help, and I was finally free of him entirely.

I always wanted to understand how my brain worked so I have always opted to not accept medication to help quieten the noise in my head. Over the years though, rehashing the same psychological issues wasn't enough for me. But I still couldn't work out why I was so different. I couldn't work out why I could remember things so vividly, like they happened yesterday. I can remember when I was a baby in nappies. I thought that was bizarre. Why could I remember things, numbers, images, places, events etc. with such clarity? How did I know things with such detail? Why did the smallest detail mean so much to me and why did it have such an impact on me when the details were omitted? Why was accuracy so important? And why could I not cope with change? I would lose my mind if things were not in the right order, and I process information, words from mouths and in written form, literally. I would struggle daily with people not comprehending that the words they used were not put into action in the manner in which they had used them. So I kept seeking different therapists throughout the course of my relationships, constantly trying to change who I was as a person, all whilst trying to fit into each relationship. And it never worked for me, or any of my relationships.

Most people think of abuse as the most common forms, emotional, psychological, physical, sexual and financial. Undoubtedly, the highest form of abuse is self-abuse. Yet it's usually the last thing anybody looks at. Am I being kind to myself by choosing this? What is the gift in creating and perpetuating this abuse? How different would this world be if inhabitants nurtured themselves? Self-abuse creates the greatest divide and separation. It's the ultimate act of withdrawal. Who you truly be is hidden from the world. The gift you are and the contribution you be gets shut off, and no two people are the same. Each of us has a unique contribution to be to the planet and universe, and to the people we choose to be a part of our lives. Even to the strangers we cross paths with, those sliding door moments, or coincidences we encounter, they are contributions. Each of those moments changes something in the universe.

Until my marriage fell apart I never really understood my place here. I had bought all my stories from the past and owned them like a badge of honour. I had grown and changed after every relationship but this was different. I remember asking my therapist during a session how was it that I could withstand so much abuse. It was like I had wired myself to accept the challenge of receiving abuse, and it was where I created the most in my life. I asked "How much abuse is one person supposed to be able to handle?!' The response surprised me; she didn't know and couldn't answer me, as she had never met anyone like me. When she thinks of me she thinks of energy, just this ball of energy, and that was her only explanation for why I could handle the level of abuse I had perpetuated throughout my lifetime.

Once I had children it became evident to me that both my kids are different. They are different to each other too, after all, aren't we all different? I knew they were autistic, but there was more to it. They each present different traits and the triggers that are consistent with both of them, trigger meltdowns in both at the same time. Being a career mother and trying to juggle my life, marriage, work, home and parenthood wore me down. I had been the emotional and psychological rock for our entire family and I couldn't continue to moderate everybody and still function. When I acknowledged this, my marriage disintegrated. As a mother I was determined to give my children more than I got. Expecting them to conform to the normalcy of this reality wasn't going to cut it for me, or them. My desire to honour who they be and to celebrate the difference they be has been one of the main drivers for how I parent my children. Trying to hammer a square peg into a round hole only succeeds in damaging the peg and the hole. It's been tough, isolating and lonely at times. Having two parents with different parenting styles has been difficult for everyone. Not a day goes by I'm not grateful for my children being who they be, and being the contribution to my life. They say they pick us, and I've finally realised why they picked me. I champion for them, teach them and lead them into a different future. I choose to be a voice for them and to help them to find their voices. I choose to raise them to follow their instincts, their gut, knowing, and awareness. I choose to show them they are a contribution and being different is to be celebrated. I choose to teach them there is nothing wrong with them, they are not faulty, if they choose to change it's for them and not by definition of others opinions of who they should and shouldn't be.

There's no parenting manual that teaches you how to parent through abuse, regardless of whether you are the perpetrator or not. Sure, there are a million books available of what parenting looks like, or should look like. All the highly recommended and most appropriate formula's and ideals to raise healthy kids but let's face it, there are a plethora of other factors that are beyond your control. Babies aren't born with an instruction book, you have no idea what this little being is going to choose or create. In our house it's very dynamic, so it happens quickly. I watch for subtle cues in changes in behaviour, facial expressions, changes in their eyes. It's the subtleties that, if missed, can escalate into a full blown meltdown and that can include throwing, punching, kicking, spitting, biting, screaming, and swearing.

It's not always ease trying to explain to people who've never had any exposure to autism, and the different traits and levels. There's a magic to my kids though, as they have capacities and abilities that far outweigh the meltdowns. It's not all they be, it's only one small component of what they have to offer, and I'm creating a future for them where they aren't defined by the supposed smallness of the disorder. They aren't defined by everything they are told they can't do or achieve.

As I move into the future creating an entirely different reality for my children, and me, I'm happier than I've ever been. My family, children and friends are valued and celebrated. There are challenges daily, it's a dynamic household with three autistics living together and it's not always ease. That's the secret to living though, the power of choice. I created this life through the choices I made, and whilst it has been filled with abuse it has also been filled with other memories. There's a quote Gary Douglas, the founder of Access Consciousness® uses often... "Never give up, never give in, never quit." It was my own personal driver long before I was introduced to the tools of Access Consciousness. I use them daily to create change, by asking questions rather than searching for answers. I do desire to live the rest of my life without abuse, that's my choice now. The challenge with balancing this is the allowance I have for my children to be who they truly be, which partly includes abusing me. We will grow together as a family and my role as a parent will in part, be fulfilled when my children surpass me in everything they choose and create.

Life is not limited to the number of checkboxes on a form. Abuse doesn't have to be a box you tick.

To anyone reading this, you are not alone. You can create something different and abuse is not all you deserve. You deserve a life of happiness and joy, filled with wide-eyed dreams. Each day you wake to the possibility of creating something new and different, and each choice, regardless of how small, is one step closer to you embracing the you you truly be. Grab it, it is right in front of you, waiting for you to unhide and choose you. Thank you, from me to you.

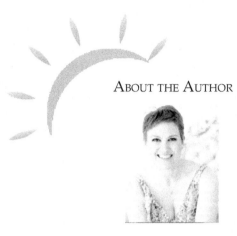

About the Author

Heather Bell

Born Heather Naomi Bell in Geelong, Victoria, Australia as the last of five children to two secondary school teachers; one just happened to also be a clergyman. Heather spent all of her first 17 years in Geelong, before embarking on an adventure to Perth and back to Melbourne, within the space of 6 months. Finally settled in Melbourne for the last 27 years, hardly settling in one spot for too long. Having moved nearly annually, Heather created a life ever changing logistically however the one constant was the capacity to sustain unhappiness, largely caused by years of ongoing abuse. Heather is different, and going undiagnosed with High Functioning Aspergers created its own challenges. Heather spent most of her life hiding who she was from everyone, as any attempt to be her was generally ridiculed, so it was easier to hide than face rejection. Making the choice to step up and be true to who you truly be has been the most challenging choice of all. The only expert on the planet, in who you are as a person and how you manage your own abuse, is you. Choosing beyond abuse is a personal choice. Heather spends her time now creating a life and living for her two autistic children by following opportunities presented (jack of all trades, master of all of them), coaching others on the crazy art of following your awareness, and being a different parent. Heather's future includes more writing, more coaching, creating a vision of a different style of parenting for neuro non-typical children, and creating a life she truly desires, all with a different perspective.

Speaking of a different perspective; Heather can be found creating different content on her Facebook page www.facebook.com/adifferentperspectivewithaccess.

Using the tools of Access Consciousness® to create change as an Access Consciousness® Bars Facilitator and running Bars® classes; Heather can be contacted via email at heather1naomi@gmail.com for Bars® appointments and/or class information, or private coaching/facilitation.

CHAPTER 13

A Whole New World

Chelsea Gibson

I woke up the other day and realized how different my life was from yesterday, a year ago, and even 10 years ago. When I wake up I don't have a judgmental person judging my body, I don't have someone telling me how wrong I am or listing off the perceived mistakes I made that day twirling in stories of mistakes years ago. I don't have to worry when I go to a change room that trying on a pair of pants that may not fit means that I am the most hideous woman in the world. There isn't worry about the physical harm that may come if I say the wrong thing or don't act perfect. What has changed? How do you go from being afraid to make a mistake or look unattractive to a world of allowance, kindness and joy? The answer isn't just breaking up with abusive people. The abusive person I needed to break up with was me.

What if the one abusive person you've never fired was internal? What if one of the unkind people to you is you? If that is the case for you or someone else I invite you to a totally inconceivable reality. That is a reality beyond making you wrong and abuse.

The most dynamic changes in my life have occurred when I stopped making myself wrong. If I can do this, so can you. A new dawn is breaking… is now the time to end the abuse with you?

An Aware Girl in a Judgmental World

In my last publication, *The Energy of Play*, I went into detail about my upbringing as a playful girl in a serious world. I was a very aware child and much of my childhood was spent in attempts to facilitate the overwhelming amount of information coming my way. I was a gifted healer and had natural sensitivities to people's pains and had a desire to help. I was sensitive to all stimuli including physical sensations as well as emotional. Everything was processed with a level of intensity. That did not stop or diminish my ability to have my reality. My reality at its core was based in joy, curiosity, play and no judgment. There is a key piece missing to a child who is 1. Aware and 2. Lives in a reality that does not match the world. It is the ability to know and differentiate between being aware of an external world and the world the child lives in. Through the mist of awareness's, thoughts and emotions, an aware child can have a difficult time separating what is theirs and what is someone or something else's. A particular energy that had the most dynamic affect on my ability to function was judgment.

To a child with little points of views, judgment can feel like daggers. In this culture children aren't taught to receive. Many families don't talk about how to receive a gift, receive a compliment, receive money and most don't talk about how to receive judgment. Since the world we raise our children in is based in wrong and right a child who tends to internally judge more than externally takes judgment as a score against themselves every time they perceive it. Therefore an aware child, brought up in a world of judgment learns quickly that their reality of is wrong and the child starts to mimic the judgment they perceive around them. That is where my story of self-abuse begins.

For example, I had an older sister that was the epitome of feminine embodiment. I on the other hand was an eccentric child, who spoke her mind, was philosophical, goofy and couldn't compute gender roles. I was aware of the judgments of right (my feminine sister) and wrong (me, the child who didn't fit in a box). It wasn't that I didn't just fit in the girl box; I didn't fit in any box. As I became increasingly aware of societal norms, I began at a very young age to judge my body, to judge my intellect and to judge my very being. Until the age of 30 I thought my body was wrong because it didn't look like the epitome of a feminine body, although the truth is that there is no right or wrong body. Gary Douglas of Access Consciousness once said to me "there is a bum for every seat". Who knew all I had to do was choose people who liked my body rather than chasing after validation from people who would judge it.

As a teenager the external reality imbedded itself into my internal reality which began poisoning the joy, the kindness and the place of no judgment. As I perceived the judgment in the world, as I got older I started buying it as real and thus I began to judge myself with it. The first time I attempted to harm myself was at the age of fourteen because I just didn't want to be that sensitive anymore. I didn't realize that I had the power to create a reality beyond the external environment. I didn't realize the awareness and the difference that I judged myself with was actually what the world required.

Where is my Mind?

When a dramatic event at a party at the age of 17 led to a rape, a pregnancy, and eventually, the loss of the baby at the beginning of my first year in college, my internal judgment increased tremendously.

I could not forgive myself. I had an internal hatred that became the foundation of how I treated myself and how I allowed others to treat me. Regardless of the support of my family and friends I retracted from everyone who cared about me to the arms of an abusive boyfriend who would abuse me externally the way I abused myself internally.

Even after leaving him I spent years in avoidance, not being present and in a constant state of wrongness and guilt. I recall moments where I couldn't breathe without thinking "Do I look fat?" It didn't matter how skinny I got or what make up I wore, there was judgment. I had no pragmatic awareness of what was true, what was a projection and what was my reality. If I made a mistake I was the worst person to exist. My true viewpoint would come in and out in fragments while waves of self-abuse crashed in the wake. I became a master of hiding my despair until another abusive situation would unearth all the internal hatred.

My reality was very distorted. Mistakes were drastic examples of how wrong I was, not fitting in a pair of pants meant I was horribly unattractive and being different than what was normal... was possibility the worst offense of all. This invalidated my very being, making it difficult to receive kindness, compliments and choosing a partner who would be fun and kind. If this is you, know you're not alone. Your reality is there somewhere amidst the emotions, thoughts and darkness. What if there was a way you could tell what was true for you, beyond others points of reference? What if there was a way you could have your reality while being in allowance of what you perceive in the world?

What is Judgment?

How much of your life do you spend doing judgment rather than living? One definition of a judge is *"a person appointed to decide in any competition, contest or matter at issues; authorized arbiter."* By this definition you've made yourself the appointed official of your life to continuously arbitrate you in relation to the world. This requires you to compete with everyone and everything during every moment. Therefore to get you out of judgment of yourself requires you to change your role in your life.

Why am I talking about self-judgment in a compilation book about breaking up with abuse? It's because there is a direct correlation between the way my life looked when I judged myself incessantly and now that I don't. In my experience, the atrocious way I treated myself created the perfect environment for external abuse to exist. When the internal environment of self-hatred and self-abuse changed, the way I interacted with the world changed. The world wasn't scary and I was not a victim.

Ending Self-Judgment

Welcome to a whole new way of being in the world. What would your life look like if you didn't judge you? Since getting out of judgment of me I have a sense of ease with my body, mental states and I have created a life I love to live. I'm not afraid of being wrong, not looking perfect. While working out and eating is fun, making mistakes can be FUN! This way of being has created a life beyond abuse.

Judgment as a way of living was not working for me. That inner spark I naturally have that is not willing to give up or give in was what kept me alive through all of the abuse. Deep down in every dark moment of receiving abuse I knew that this was not why I was on the planet. I knew there must be more to life than me spending every moment judging me.

Today I am thankful for Cognitive Behavioral Therapy, which was the beginning to change my inner thoughts with the help of a meditation practice I had as a child. I am thankful for the tools of Access Consciousness and its founder Gary Douglas which I found at the age of twenty-eight. Who knew that same awareness that created the judgment in my world was the same awareness that led me to a workshop in Amsterdam that I knew nothing about and that changed my life forever?

Judgment is such a normal phenomenon on this planet, which is why it becomes normal so early in our lives. Where did you learn judgment? Let's create a mental environment for you where judgment seems silly and ridiculous rather than normal. Once you stop making judgment valuable, you can start to unravel the wrongness you believe you are and begin to be nurturing and kind to you. In turn, you start choosing a life beyond abuse.

You are like this beautiful piano that can be played. If you don't have the keys of self-judgment, another person can't play the notes of abuse because they aren't there. You will confuse and possibly frustrate abusive people because they can't play the song of abuse to you. You begin to function from this place where you can receive their viewpoint or their actions and it doesn't feel like a dagger. It can be about asking you questions "What is this pain or emotion I am aware of?".

You can be aware "wow this is unkind" and then ask "now what can I choose?" At the point you become aware that someone is judging you or being unkind, you have choice. You may choose to break up with them, choose a different job, or say something. The point is, you are not a victim. You have total choice and with allowance, this is a potion for a reality that once was inconceivable to you. Once I realized that I wasn't this awful person, I could have my back. If you choose to have your back from a place of no judgment and awareness, you can choose in any moment what you'd like to create. If something isn't working, choose to create something different or be the difference that invites people to change.

"How would you be if you could perceive you without judgment?" According to Dr. Dain Heer, it is more about the demand of yourself for yourself to be out of judgment of you, starting today. Regardless of your body weight, size, money, job, status, relationships, etc. This is the most important key to ending abuse. You must start to demand that you get out of judgment of yourself and be present with that every moment of everyday. When you start to do that, abuse will not be an acceptable behavior in your world.

One of the greatest ways people manipulate and abuse is through guilt and shame. When you don't build your life on whether you are right or wrong people can't guilt or shame you. It is just their interpretation of what occurred and you can have your own. You can also be the kindness to you that you have been hoping and wishing someone else to be. I could not receive the amount of kindness today if it weren't for me being totally kind to me. It's the same as not being able to receive a compliment when you don't think it's true for you. When I am kind to myself and really see my beauty, I can receive all kinds of praise, compliments, sex, joy, playfulness, money, fun and experiences. I get to explore the world through playing with it because I am not wrong if I make a mistake. I am just learning!

You and your reality is in there somewhere. Through the abuse, through the judgment and through the confusion YOU are there. There is a spark inside you that nobody can take away or kill or abuse out of you. If you find that, nurture it and are kind to it you'll find it will be the dawn of your new day.

About the Author

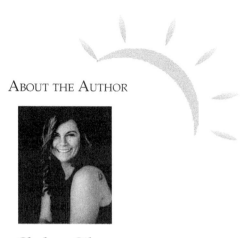

Chelsea Gibson

Chelsea Gibson is a #1 international bestselling author, the CEO of Wild Rose Wellness, and is a Cognitive Behavior Therapist, Access® Bars Facilitator and Energetic Facilitator. Through her own evolution mentally and spiritually Chelsea realized her childhood passion for energy, meditation and helping people was reignited through her Business. Chelsea has continued to travel around the world learning different tools in Access Consciousness, meditation, spiritual traditions, workshops and tools for a happier and healthier life to be able to provide a wide variety of services and perspectives for her clients. She now provides private sessions as well as teaches workshops and certifications in a variety of modalities and topics in the hopes of facilitating people on being more playful with creating their lives and bodies. Chelsea has an energy that is addictive to be around. Just try to not smile and laugh with this potent and bubbly being! Don't be fooled, when push comes to shove Chelsea will be able to blast your limitations and expectations away. She is gifted with helping people get to know their own bodies, and get into joyful communion with them. You can find her at www.WildRoseWellness.net.

CHAPTER 14

Breaking Up is Magic Too!

Margriet Emerick

The relationship I talk of was undoubtedly abusive but it was also an essential part of my soul dance in this lifetime.

A healer priest told me much later I had always been destined to go to Bali but in the end it didn't happen till I was 36. I was hardly young but it felt like I was, just divorced after a long marriage.

I went reluctantly having no interest in Indonesia but just out of convenience, initially only for a quick holiday to a cheap place. Later only did I know just what a major part Bali would play in my life.

There's no need for me to give you all the details of how we met, I will try to focus on just how over time, the breakup from that relationship took place.

Ubud, Bali was the romantic setting for it all. A motor bike was the usual transport. My relationship was with an unlikely man, a womaniser, a flirt, a storyteller and singer, full of jokes and hugs. Not handsome at all but the rest made up for it.

At the beginning, it was full of the usual Balinese romantic experiences. Having dinner in little lamp lit warungs, riding around on the back of a motor bike along little roads flanked by brilliant green rice fields, bathing in cool village springs in the hills, being taken as a villager to traditional dances and gamelan performances and lots of love making. So it went on for about three months. We had plenty of time. I had come back on a leisurely yearlong trip on leave from my job.

While fully engrossed in this new romance, entered into with many misgivings that had to be put aside, and overcome by the excitement of the affair, something happened of great significance.

Rather strangely one night I was alone, having dinner at a little warung in Ubud when mid-meal I suddenly felt a strong urge to go back to my room in the small palace where I stayed. The feeling became irresistible so I left my meal, paid hurriedly and, through dark streets, walked as quickly as I could as if drawn by a magnetic force.

Back in my room I closed the old Bali style divided door and bolted it with the wooden bolt and lay on my bed wondering what was happening. I soon realised that I was unable to move and was immobilised on the bed. After a while I gradually realised that I was not alone.

For those that don't (yet) believe in a spirit world inhabited by spirits, let me just say that an energy force was present diagonally across from my bed in the corner of the room. It was more than 3 metres in height and surmounted by an energetic face of a fierce black male. Of the body I perceived little but perhaps a traditional chequered black and white cloth. Telepathically the force spoke to me giving me a stern warning.

The warning was about my lover, about his intentions and hidden motivations and the follow-up was that I must stop the relationship immediately.

I stood my ground and said that was impossible, that I loved him and nothing could change that! Even as I thought it, I was amazed at my audacity and courage. The thought of my foolhardiness did not occur to me unfortunately. I could have explored the meaning of the warning and asked questions but that also did not occur to me.

In fact, I was still immobile on the bed and stayed that way for a few hours. Gradually the ability of being able to move came back and I was able to sob and express my fright. At about midnight I got up, looked around and saw nothing but was still badly shaken and frightened. But not frightened enough as it turned out…

The next morning, I was conscious of a very bad smell around my room. When my breakfast came I mentioned it and asked for a special thorough cleaning of my bathroom as that seemed to be where the smell was strongest.

The cleaner came and scrubbed everywhere with strong bleach but still the putrid smell remained. The owner's mother came later and asked if I could still smell it and when I said I could, she returned with the cleaner and scrubbed everything again. It made no difference at all, but over the next few days the smell gradually disappeared. No one was surprised by it and they seemed to accept that I had had a visitation from a being from another spiritual dimension and the lingering smell was the common sign of that.

My Bali relationship continued unabated for the rest of the year and on for another 11 years. Events included my resignation from my job, my relocation to various teaching jobs in Bali and other parts of Indonesia, Post Graduate study in Sydney, and my search for ways that would allow me to live in Bali and somehow earn a living to support myself and satisfy the demands for financial support from my partner.

While I was in Sydney, my partner made a one-month visit there. It was difficult for us both as he came in between Balinese festivals and that coincided with the most demanding parts of my study year and the work I was doing to support us. He spent many days either entertaining other Balinese friends in Sydney to coffee and kretek cigarette gatherings at my lodgings or on lone sight seeing trips around the city.

One of the highlights for him was visiting building sites and seeing the local Australians working at menial labouring jobs. He found it hard to believe what he saw. It was something that had never occurred to him, that in their own country it would be them doing the hard work. It was such a contrast to how he saw them on holiday in Bali, lounging by swimming pools or being driven around to see the sights.

During this time, I endured years of intermittent happiness and despair, learning to live with his unfaithfulness, his lies and evasiveness, his gambling and the incessant demands for money to support this habit when at times I hardly knew when my next dollar was coming from and I had a zero bank balance. It was counterbalanced of course by his charm, warmth and humor or I guess I couldn't have stayed in the relationship.

At the end of 11 years, I was living in another village a few kilometers south of Ubud. I had set up a small business making handmade paper and stationery, books and other items from the paper and other locally available natural materials like banana bark. I had done this originally as a way to support myself and still stay in Bali near my loved one.

Since I had so little money the business was miraculously set up with a working capital of $300 and amazingly it worked. Supportive boutique hotels and curious designers looking for new products helped us and each month, though it was tight, we managed to find enough income to survive on and to pay the wages of half a dozen staff.

It was late afternoon and every one had gone home for the day when I heard the sound of the Kawasaki motorbike pulling up outside the building I rented as both office and workspace, and home. So much had passed between us, so much hurt and struggle, my heart no longer felt any excitement at hearing it. I just felt the dull expectation of hearing more demands on me, for money and help that I was little equipped to provide.

We greeted each other in the office and I left the computer where I'd been entering data and went with him into the living room. I could see from the distant look on his face and the dark flush on his skin, that he had come from some more engrossing activity, most probably cock fighting or playing cards, to see me. That meant only one thing - he needed money. That could be the only possible explanation for him to interrupt his favourite activity.

As he moved to take me in his arms, a vision of a long tunnel cave formed in my head. I saw it stretching into the future and into infinite time. I saw my life and his, until the time of death and beyond, over and over, going through the same quarrels and making up that usually made up our days.

According to one of his stories, in my last lifetime, after death when I wanted to cross the Bardo, the bridge in Balinese legend, he had carried me as I couldn't cross it by myself. That was the reason I had stayed so resolutely in my relationship with him in this lifetime, in order to repay him for the service he had performed for me then in the afterlife.

The energy of what I saw in the tunnel built up, I saw the seesawing of our relationship, the highs and the lows being repeated to infinity. I saw the petty hurts and humiliations repeating, in between them the passion and love, the demands for money, the lies and avoidances of the addicted gambler.

And suddenly it seemed totally ridiculous to me that I had stayed with it for so long in this prison of love. In an instant I saw that this wasn't love or at least it wasn't the type of love that I wanted. Involuntarily I started to laugh at the ridiculousness of it all, and as I laughed, the walls of my relationship prison started to shake, to crack and then to slowly melt away,

The effect on him was instantaneous. He stood there looking foolish, not angry but stunned into silence for a while. Unusual for him, and yet giving room for the breaking of the spell between us. There was no anger just a momentous change in the energy between us that was impossible to ever undo.

Slowly with a muted goodbye, he left the room, started his bike, got on and rode slowly away.

I wondered in the shock of it all, what I had done. Would I ever see him again? I thought it unlikely and, at the same time as feeling free, I felt sad as well.

I needn't have worried. Within a few days he was back visiting again but from this day on, as my friend. No demands, no more love affair, just a warm and devoted friend. That is the way it remained until he died.

I was so grateful that I had been able to summon the energy to change our relationship. The laughter turned out to be the magic that was required to shatter the spell that I had been under for all those years. In an instant it shattered the intense emotional energy that had been my bond for so long. I could see clearly which way my suffering ended and my freedom lay.

In an instant we became close in a way that we had never been before. There was no more manipulative behaviour. Honesty, vulnerability and openness was possible as it never had before.

This man was a delightful friend as I had seen all along that he was to the other people of his village and to other foreigners. He was entertaining and caring, a great story teller and raconteur. He sang funny old songs and he told the traditional Balinese stories in endlessly entertaining ways. He accompanied me with groups of friends to holy springs and to ancient temples. He listened to me when I needed to talk.

Of course these were all things that he had been all along. It was just that as the years passed, I saw them less and less in what had been a struggle for domination in our relationship.

He was heavy of foot, deep of voice, and had a great sense of humor. He was not a violent man. The hardships of his childhood when he and his family had almost starved in famines and rat plagues left him unable to feel the struggles of others. That is what I had never realised. For him, asking and receiving for whatever he needed was the normal way of life.

In not listening to the powerful warning I was given almost at the beginning of our relationship, I had ensured that I would remain in Bali for many years to come. Did that serve me well? Strangely I believe that it did. In the midst of great despair comes spiritual awakening, I have found. So I will always be grateful for the good times that we shared and in retrospect, I can accept the less happy times as well.

Another man may not have reacted in the same way to my laughter but for us the time had come to break up. The impossible situation for me had to come to an end. Although I didn't consciously choose to laugh, that was what turned out to be instrumental in breaking us apart.

Do I have any advice for others? I don't think I do. For every one of us is different and every relationship is different. Don't necessarily listen to advice from others, even if they are more than 3 meters high, but know yourself and listen to your spirit and your body. If it wants to be free, it will find a way. That's part of the magic of life and living!

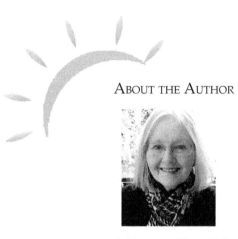

ABOUT THE AUTHOR

Margriet Emerick

Margriet Emerick was born in Australia but has enjoyed living in Indonesia, mostly in Ubud on the island of Bali, for over 35 years. During this time she has been a university lecturer and a trained counsellor and, as you would expect, many other things as well.

On the slopes of the volcano Gunung Agung at a small temple a few meters from Pura Besakih, the mother temple of Balinese Hinduism, she became a Balinese Tapakan intuitive healer about twenty years ago and was given the Balinese name of Jero Gingsir. It was most unexpected and came like a bolt of lightning! She studied with a Pemangku priest healer over several years, and later underwent further purification and consecration ceremonies from a Pedanda or Brahman High Priestess.

The Balinese rituals and teachings awakened a curiousity in her about other cultures' healing techniques and in later years, she studied several including Mayan Light Language and more recently Access Consciousness™. She is now an Certified Access Bars Facilitator™ and an Access Body Process Facilitator™ , as well as an Intuitive Counsellor and is available for client sessions in Bali, or in Canberra, Australia or through the Internet.

She also found a new calling as a designer of Soul Jewelry, using images that speak to the spirit and, with the help of Bali's highly skilled traditional village carvers and silversmiths, turns them into beautiful and unique jewelry which is available to order both retail and wholesale, either from her website or as a Custom order by email.

You can learn more about Margriet at:
    www.margrietemerick.accessconsciousness.com
    www.kertasgingsir.com

Please contact Margriet at: gingsir@gmail.com.

Chapter 15

Relationships - Food for Your Soul

Jeneen Yungwirth

Relationship is simply one area of your life, there are also other areas as well. Finances, health, and career for example. One thing I teach all of my clients and students is that you cannot separate these from one another. It is like having a peeing section in a pool. It just doesn't work. So if you have issues in one or more of these areas of your life, they are all affecting one another because they run together. They are all a part of you. My target for this chapter for you is to gain some different insights into what relationships are and can be for you, as well as to offer you some tools for creating change in this area of your life if you are willing to know that things can change!

I have had a very interesting take on relationships for my entire life. I require ease in relationships and prefer not to have drama. It wasn't until recently that I actually acknowledged I might have a capacity for creating ease in my life with relationships! Now it hasn't always been easy per say, and yet somehow I create ease for myself. There may be some concepts here that are going to be really out there and you have to take what works for you. But if you are looking for change and more ease in this area of your life, it might be something you want to keep open to as you read through what I have to say.

Self Care – The most important relationship you will have - is the relationship you have with yourself. I work with so many clients and people who come to my group readings who don't know what self-care is. They have forgotten themselves somewhere in the mix of life and many people are feeling empty and depleted. Many people think that self-care is selfish. What if I were to tell you that you are the only one who knows exactly what you require? Do you know what they tell you on an airplane when the oxygen masks come down? They tell you to put your mask on before assisting others! Is this selfish? We die without oxygen. Do you know that many people are running out of air because they are not looking out for their needs? They think they have to assist others before they can get to what is important for them. So many people are feeling depleted and guess what? You cannot give from an empty vessel.

We know that food is what nurtures the physical body, so what if relationships are the food for your soul? Consider this. When you go to a buffet what do you eat? What you feel like eating that day or do you choose to eat foods you don't like and that make your tummy hurt? Seems like a silly question right? What if relationships are the same? What if one day you like chicken but the next you prefer steak? Is that wrong?

We are energy. Period. We all evolve at different rates. There is no right or wrong here. When we meet people at a period in our lives, we are at a certain vibration. This energy of who we be involves our dreams, our interests and whatever stage of life we are at. So when you meet these people and you hit it off it simply means you have lots in common and similar interests. As the years go by you evolve and your interests change and so do theirs. Sometimes you no longer have as much in common, it is natural, things change over time. Does it make it right or wrong? Nope, people change, situations change and circumstances change. Change is the one constant in this world.

Now as I said earlier, relationships are about what nurtures you as a being. I have many friendships that I have had for years and to this day, months can go by and if we run into one another or call it is like no time has passed. There are no judgments or expectations. Simply acceptance. Those are the relationships that work for me.

I recently had to break off a friendship. It was someone I became friends with in Business College. We met before we had children – she wasn't married yet. It was somewhat of a needy friendship in the beginning as she had no siblings and she thought of me like a sister. I am very independent and love my space. Again no right here no wrong, we all have different requirements. It is important to acknowledge what works for each person as an individual. There were times where we spent all day together at college and then I would get home and she would call in the evening. At times I would get frustrated, as I just wanted to spend time with my husband. Young and not wanting to be rude, I never said anything. Already there were parts of the relationship that weren't working for me.

As the years went on she got married, then I had children and a few years after that she then had children also. I got busier and busier as I added a couple of businesses into the mix and started to meet more and more people who were interested in the same things I was interested in. Time went on and I changed – a lot! I was doing a lot of self-discovery and looking into transformational therapies. It became a huge part of my life. I also was very busy, and really didn't have a lot of time for socializing anymore with kids and work. Which really worked for my husband and I and our family. Unfortunately, it didn't work for the friendship and she was very disappointed. I knew it hurt her to not see me but a few times a year. I tried talking with her and to get her to open up about it and she wouldn't say anything to me. It was then that I knew it wasn't going to work anymore. Each time I did see her all I could sense was disappointment and a lot of judgment instead of gratitude for the time we did get to have together. Now here is where it gets really interesting and I learned a lot.

I couldn't quite pin point why the relationship wasn't working anymore, it just felt sort of toxic to me. Even though I was trying to make it work, she simply wasn't happy with how the friendship was anymore. Each time I would get together with her I would either get angry or really ill. I couldn't figure out what was wrong with me. Looking back now I think it is funny that I thought something was wrong with me, when really I was picking up on how she was feeling. One day we were grocery shopping and I suddenly started to feel ill again. I told my husband we needed to hurry up because I wasn't feeling well and needed to get home to bed. My head was throbbing. A few moments later guess who we ran into? She was in the store and what was really interesting to me was my body knew it before my cognitive mind knew it.

I decided I really needed to ask myself if the relationship with her was nurturing for me anymore? In a word, no. Does that mean it was wrong or bad? Not at all. It is simply a choice. So what if every relationship in your life was simply a choice. Just like going to the buffet. If you went to the same buffet every week, you might choose some things over and over again because you enjoy them so much and other things you might switch up simply because you wanted or required something else that day. So what if your relationships could be the same? Just a choice as you evolve and they evolve. If one day you wake up and it no longer works for you what if you could simply choose something else?

The definition of relationship is the distance between two objects.

Communication – I don't want you to get me wrong here. You MUST communicate with all of your relationships. You can't just read this chapter and then break up with all of the relationships that aren't working for you! It is important to know you must have some conversations with these people to see if the relationship is salvageable? Is one of you or both ready to move on? As I mentioned I tried talking to my friend on a few occasions and she wouldn't open up when I would bring it up.

Any relationships that have been difficult in my life there have been conversations. In each of them I have been willing to talk about what is working and what isn't working. If they are unwilling to look at the things I bring up (and they also have the freedom to express how they feel about the relationship as well, it is give and take after all) then I make a decision as to if it will continue or if I have to let it go.

Holding on to old toxic relationships doesn't allow for new ones to come to our lives as we evolve and change. It is like having full closets, where are you going to put the new stuff? I call it cleaning out the relationship closet. We are all individuals with unique requirements of what works for you - and you must listen to what works for you. You must also get that people will treat us how we let them. Each time I had a visit with this friend all I got from her was hurt and disappointment with how she felt about our friendship, and that no longer worked for me. It was no longer nurturing. I had to let it go.

How to clean out the relationship closet – The natural evolution of friendships will often just peter out on their own. Especially when we are young because we tend to make relationships much less significant. Somewhere as we get older we think we have to be loyal, etc. What if it is just an evolution of letting go and more and more time goes between visits? I tried this in this relationship yet she was unwilling to let me go and at the same time when we saw each other she couldn't hide her disappointment with how it was.

Marriage - I must say that I feel very lucky to have an amazing relationship with my husband. I also acknowledge that going into this relationship I knew myself well enough to know what I required in a relationship. To be honest I thought I was too picky and that I would never get married!! I had dated several other people and ended up breaking up with them because they just weren't a match. I couldn't imagine waking up to their face every single day! This may sound rude, but I knew what I required and was looking for in a relationship if I was going to be happy! I figured I was much too picky and it wouldn't happen. We have now been happily married for 22 years and I love him more today than the day I married him. We support each other. It hasn't always been easy and there have been some serious conversations as I expressed what I required in the relationship. Communication from day one has been of utmost importance as we have moved through the years. It wasn't always easy for him to express himself but I wouldn't take that in the relationship. There were times where I would put all of my thoughts, feelings and emotions out on the table and he would sit quiet. I would have to coax it out of him explaining to him that he now had the whole story and I only had half. Mine! So I had to really encourage him to open up to me. Something he wasn't used to as he didn't see this growing up in his family. Be the space of allowance for your partner to be vulnerable, as I was. I let him know I wanted to know what he thought. It was ok for him to express himself. I was willing to change or look at his point of view and see where we could improve if required, that it was important to express what was important to him as well.

5 Tools for creating more ease in all of your relationships!

I love using the tools of Access Consciousness.

#1 One of the things I learned here is that whatever is light for you is true for you and if something is heavy it is either a lie or not true for you. This gives you freedom in your choices. What I love about following this energy of light vs. heavy is you don't have to figure everything out, your awareness will guide you!

There have been times where it is heavy to answer the phone when someone is calling me. Either I am just not the one with the information they are looking to pull out of me (those relationships that are energy suckers), or maybe it just isn't the right time for the reason they are calling. Invited to an event or party? Not sure you want to go? Follow if it is light or heavy for you.

#2 Asking questions to gain awareness. What is right about me that I am not getting or seeing? Asking a question will always bring more awareness! It isn't about getting an answer either; you will get awareness's. So earlier I said one of the most important relationships you will ever have is with yourself! We judge ourselves at times more than others judge us. So are you willing to stop judging you and ask what is right about you? We all have weaknesses, and that is not where our attention should be! Also how many judgments are you aware of from others that you have bought as true? We can't be good at everything! What we are looking for is our strengths and it is time for you to acknowledge yours! You could also ask what are my strengths? What am I good at? Are there strongnesses that you have that you have made a wrongness? For example, I used to think my impatience was a wrongness and that I needed to learn patience. I now realize that I actually have a capacity to get things done efficiently and effectively. I have also learned that

I am not willing to settle because I know there are better ways of getting things done or getting the results that I know are possible!

#3 Destroy and Uncreate your relationships every day. This allows all of your points of view to be erased about everything you believe your relationship to be or not be. This allows the space of something else to be possible. This helps to take you out of the judgment of the relationship as well. How do you destroy and uncreate your relationships? Simply say everything I've decided my relationship is or isn't I destroy and uncreate it all!

#4 Show me what I truly desire in my relationships? Asking this question will help you get awareness on what works for you and may open doors to the possibilities for what you would like to create moving forward with your relationships.

#5 What would it take to have more ease, joy and glory in all of my relationships? Ask this every day especially if relationships are a challenge in your life...

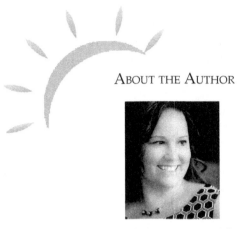

About the Author

Jeneen Yungwirth

Jeneen Yungwirth is an author, speaker and radio show host on A2Zen.fm. Her radio show is Just Show Up with Jeneen. Jeneen has been studying transformational energy for nearly 15 years and has played with numerous tools for creating change, ease and joy in her own personal life as well as working with groups through classes and one on one in private sessions. The only way she can describe some of the change she has witnessed for herself and her clients is magical. Jeneen teaches that you are the creator of your life and if something isn't working for you she empowers you with the tools to change it. Changing energy and lives with these simple tools is beyond miraculous in her eyes and magical seems to fit so much more. Jeneen also has the capacity as a psychic medium to connect with energies on the other side. Check out Jeneen's Facebook page Access Jeneen.

Jeneen is also the author of the book - *You Are Not Alone* - A personal journey into mediumship and connecting with the other side.

Photo credits to Hayley Porteous Flair Studios Photography

CHAPTER 16

Don't Let the Blonde Hair and Pink Nails Fool Ya!
I'm smarter and tougher than you think!

Denise Dominguez

For years and years, I was so afraid to leave my marriage. I had every excuse I could drum up; How would I make on my own (financially), what will my kids think of me leaving their dad, where would my kids and I live?

You see from the outside view, we looked like we had it all! The big house, pool, nice cars and we traveled all around the state we lived in (Florida). We looked like your average ordinary middle class happy family. Loving couple, two kids, one dog and one cat.

But that was what we looked like from the outside. On the inside there was chaos, drama, debt, arguing, metal abuse, emotional abuse, addiction, and attempted suicide – just to name a few. I was trying my best to keep our family together, never thinking of myself and what the consequences would be to my children and I. But with each passing day it got worse and worse. It seemed like the harder I tried the worse it got.

When my husband and I married in 1991 I was head over heels with this man! I vowed to myself that day that this would be the only time I ever get married and no matter what (with the exception of physical abuse and cheating), I would stay married and any obstacles in our way we would work it out. And I meant it! I was in this for the long haul, and when we had children this promise to myself meant even more to me. We are a family now and that bonds us together for life. I wanted this life, I wanted to be a wife and mom, I embraced everything that meant to my core being. I was a devoted wife to him and a devoted mom to my children. I was in love with them and would do anything for them. Life was great in the beginning. We bought our first house just before our daughter was born, my husband wanted her to come "home" and he busted his ass to make sure that that happened. When our daughter was just three months old I was pregnant again. This time we were having a baby boy. We lived a simple life. He was the provider and I was the stay at home mom. We were creating a dream life of having a family, being in love, and enjoying our kids.

Living in Florida we were able to do so much all year long like BBQs on the weekends, spending time with our family and friends, and going to Orlando often. Ahhhh…those were the good old days.

But as life got to be more of life it was slowly weighing on us as a couple.

We outgrew that house and bought a bigger one with a pool when our kids were just two and three years old. This one was a four bedroom, two car garage with a pool home on a cul-de-sac street in suburbia USA. I remember when we moved in, I felt like I was out of my league there. This neighborhood was NICE! Every lawn was immaculate, every house was very well taken care of, they all drove nice cars. There's an elementary school two blocks away. WHOA this is not where I come from but it was what we wanted for our kids, the kind of neighbor-hood you see on T.V. where people wave hello to you even if they don't know you. Just an all-around delightful area.

We lived in this house for nearly ten years and this is when our lives started to take a turn for the worse. I was approaching thirty years old and asking myself what was my purpose in life? Who am I? Yes, I am their mom and his wife, but I had an identity before them. So who am I now? I didn't have the an-swers to these questions. This was the beginning of me feeling lost in life. During this time, I was more and more dependent on my husband financially and I was putting up with more and more of his shit. I tested positive for an STD for the third time in my life and all three times were when I was married. This first time was in my first trimester of my first pregnancy with our daughter, the second time was in my first trimester with our son and the third time was about nine years later. I ignored the truth of this because if I were to face the truth I knew what I would need to do; take our kids and leave him. I didn't want our family to break up so I dismissed this as a mistake. Correc-tion; three mistakes, three separate times.

I noticed that he was sleeping more and dozing off while in a conversation with us and he would start talking randomly almost like when you talk in your sleep. Mumbling. Again I ignored all of these red flags, I ignored that his watch alarm would go off every four hours and he would take a pill. I never asked what he was taking, I never questioned him at all really, I knew what I would find out if I probed. I knew the truth but I was so good at pushing so far back in my head and solely focus on raising our family.

We always got into arguments and sometimes it got physical, but as time went on it got worse. He would get angry over the stupidest things and we would go days even weeks with-out speaking to each other. He would yell at me and even call me "fucking bitch" in front of people. This infuriated me and I would address it to him but it was a waste of time. He dismissed me as a person, so many times he cheated on me, lied to me, blamed me and controlled our kids and me.

When you are in it; you don't realize how bad it is getting day by day; the abuse, control and dependency would get deeper and deeper; to the point where you are so deep in this hole that you've created that it seems impossible to climb out of it. Where do I begin? What do I do now? These are questions I asked myself and at the same time I asked myself how can I fix this? How can I fix him?

Finally, in 2008, after we had decided to leave our newly built four-bedroom, three-bath, two-car garage ranch home on 10 acres and all be together under one roof (to live in my parents' two bedroom, one bath home), this was when the shit really hit the fan! He had been on steroids for some time now and that means getting angry and aggressive over nothing, it means being at the gym for hours and hours it also means he was getting attention from other women and he indulged in this. If you don't know about the side effects of steroids the biggest one is it brings on depression. So in addition to all of the different kinds of pills he was self-medicating himself with he was also injecting pure poison into his bloodstream and it brought on depression so fast and so deep.

It was just another crazy argument we had been in and by this time we had been married about sixteen years and our seventeenth anniversary was upon us. I was much older now and had been putting up with his crazy and controlling behavior for years now. I was so done with this life. Every day was a struggle, we never knew what mood he would be in, we constantly walked on egg shells around him.

We were no longer in love, we didn't laugh together anymore, I was realizing more and more that this wasn't going to be a "happily ever after" kind of story. And no matter what I did to try to save this marriage or save him, it was not going to happen the only person I can save now is me.

So when I was finally fed up with his bullshit and told him (again) that I wanted a divorce he tried to overdose on pills and attempted suicide by shooting himself with our fourteen-year-old daughter in the next room. You would think that this would have been the icing on the cake and I would leave him but it wasn't over yet. I was still trying to save our family. How could I leave now? My kids were now traumatized by seeing their dad on the floor with blood all around him, they felt so bad for him they knew he is sick. No one tries to take their life unless they are so submerged in their own pain and they just can't take it anymore. This is what they saw in their father, pain, loneliness, and desperation. I felt if I had left him then that I was being cold and cruel. I stayed and tried once again to mend the pieces back together. I dragged him to every mental health place that the hospital was recommending, every doctor's appointment and every psychologist in the surrounding area of where we lived. Nothing worked, nothing was sticking he was so far deep into his pain and suffering that he couldn't see the light and I was more lost than ever. I remember one time our kids and I were driving around looking for him and I saw a homeless man and I thought "that is going to be my husband" I could see him being that lost, we were all lost at this time. None of us knew what was next. I remember the two us of just crying in each other's arm's just because of the pain that we were in. We said nothing to each other we just cried. I was crying for him, I was crying for my kids and I was crying for me. Slowly he came around and we were trying to work on things.

A few years had passed by and it was December 2010 after I had gone on a weekend visit to NC to surprise my best friend on her 40th birthday. My daughter came to me and said "Mom, I don't want to go college in Florida, I want to go to college in

NC." Well...at this point we were all numb from everything that happened. We were not the same none of us. Time was just passing, I was running his appliance service business, the kids were going to school and he was running the service calls. We tried to expand the business and it was working for a while but he was still on drugs. So as fast as we gain customers and hired one, two and three new technicians, it all came crashing down. You can't be on drugs and run a business at the same time. They were stealing from us and he was getting into physical fights with these guys right there at home, in front of our kids. The crazy continues.

After my daughter said this to me I asked her to give me a few months to make a plan, and I did. I made a 6-month plan figuring we could leave in June. My plans were pushed up when my son overheard me talking about leaving and told his dad what he heard. My husband was devastated! He was hysterically crying and saying "please don't leave, please!" How could I leave him now, I asked? Once again I felt sorry for him and agreed to stay and try to work things out. Before I knew it, he had decided to go cold turkey and stop self-medicating himself to prove to me that he wasn't on anything. This led to him hallucinating every night for the next four nights. While we were all supposed to be sleeping he was hearing voices and talking to them. Yes, this actually happened. I wish I was making this shit up but I'm not. So obviously I couldn't sleep. I had to make sure he wouldn't hurt himself or leave the house or whatever. I stayed up all night long while he was hallucinating and in the morning, he didn't remember a thing. I remember asking him "How did you sleep?" and he replied "Fine." I asked, "You don't remember saying this and saying that?" He looked at me like I was the crazy one.

On the fifth morning he dosed off to sleep for a moment. I was so scared that he would stop breathing and I was constantly checking on him to make sure he was okay. His breathing was so shallow and before I knew it, he was unresponsive. I was straddled on top of him shaking him, pinching him, and screaming WAKE UP!! WAKE UP!!! Our son came running in the room hearing the yelling and tried to wake him up with no luck. "Dad...DAD!! DAD!!! Wake up" my son said. I told my son to call 911 so he ran into the other room to call them. By this time, it was 5AM in the morning and he suddenly woke up and looked at me and said "I know that guy Joe has a crush on you" and got up, grabbed his keys and took off in his van. I was so shaken up I could hardly catch my breath. "What the hell just happened?" I asked myself over and over. Yes, this really happened. Writing this and going back to these memories; it's hard for me to believe this was our life.

The police came and we told them what happened. There wasn't much they could do since he didn't commit any crime. They did go by some of the places he stops to get coffee, but he wasn't there. I went to my friend's house that was empty to get away, take a break and get some sleep. When I woke up I had a voicemail on my phone from a friend saying she thought she saw my husband driving erratically on the sidewalk and the streets. He was still hallucinating, but was really bad now! And so the saga continues.

After many trips and calls to the local police station to get them to help me find him though the GPS on his cell phone, we managed to find out where he was. He had checked into a hotel room about 5 miles from our house. The police broke his van window to see if his guns where there. Then they busted into the hotel room, cuffed him and seized his two guns lying next to him on the bed. They took him straight to the psych ward because he was still hallucinating. By this time, it was around 5 p.m.

He was safe now. My kids and I could rest and know that their dad was okay for now. We went home and rested, none of us had had that much sleep the past week. The next morning, I called the hospital and asked if I could talk to him, they responded with "we can't connect you to anyone right now we have an emergency-a patient got physical with a nurse so no calls now!" I had this feeling that that patient was my husband. I was right. He punched a nurse in the face. Because of his erratic behavior, the psych hospital had to heavily sedate him. Not knowing what chemicals were already in his body, they transferred him to the hospital and put him on a breathing machine - just in case he stopped breathing.

My heart broke for him, but at the same time, I was fucking DONE!!! I told our son to call his dad's family to come get him - I am clocking out! I couldn't take this craziness anymore.

My determination to leave and make it on my own was overpowering my fears of how I was going to make it happen. At this point, I didn't care about the "how's" - I just had to get away from this crazy life and so I did. While this was happening, I was still continuing my plan to leave. In five months, I manifested 10k to leave Florida and move to NC. I did this without a job in either state. I sold everything of value I owned and everything he owned. I held garage sales every weekend until it was down to barely anything.

I packed and moved everything out of the house that was mine and my daughters and packed his stuff and put it all in the shed. The house was empty. All of our belongings were at my friend's townhouse and we were that much closer to peace and happiness.

We were leaving for NC in about two weeks. I was excited, happy, nervous and sad all at the same time. I was leaving my 17-year-old son behind in Florida. It was just my daughter and I moving three states away from the only life we've ever known. Our entire family resides in Florida. She was leaving her dad, brother, cousins, aunts, grandparents and friends. I was leaving my son, my mom, dad, sisters, nieces, nephews, and friends. In spite of how big of a change this was we were ready for a new life. A life with peace and happiness. A home that was "OURS" with no anxiety, no yelling, no slamming doors, a calm and peaceful home. So with the 28' Penske moving truck and car carrier on the back here we go! This felt empowering and scary all at once. I didn't know what the future held but I knew this…it was better than the past. I was determined to create a beautiful life for my daughter and I.

It wasn't long after being here in NC that I was tired of the 9 to 5 work life. I ran my ex's business successfully in Florida so I know I am an entrepreneur. I was in search of my own business I wanted that #laptoplife and I was determined to get it! I found this beautiful blonde successful business coach and got on her mailing list. She offered a 7-day video series on how to create an online business with a free coaching call after the series. Well… I never thought in a million years by the end of that call I would be putting a $700 down payment and would enter into a one-year contract that was $527 a month. WHAT?? I only made about $30K a year by myself. But I wanted this and when someone asks you what your why is and your why is stronger than it had ever been before, you leap! You just do it and trust yourself and trust the process that you are in the right place at the right time. I did it! I created an online coaching business for myself. I help women that are in that same space as I was when I was feeling lost and stuck in life. I teach women the importance of self-love, self-worth and how to change their mindset into a positive one. Everything that I needed to learn about myself I now teach that to women. I am a speaker, radio show personality, host and women's empowerment coach. I travel anywhere I want to, I take as many vacations as I want, and I am my own boss. I have finally found me and every day I live out my passions in life by helping others.

I am now in a committed relationship with a man that I am so in love with. He loves me and supports me in everything.

The relationships between my son and I are back on track, my daughter and her dad's relationship is back on track and my kid's relationship with each other has been restored and mended. I did the work on me in order to be able to help others, what a reward it is to feel this free and light. Life is so GOOD now! And it gets better and better every single day. So don't let the blonde hair and pink nails fool ya! I'm smarter and tougher than you think!

About the Author

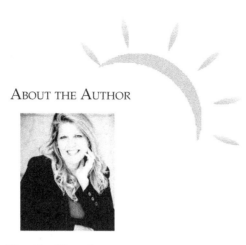

Denise Dominguez

Originally from South Florida, where she raised her two children, Denise Dominguez is a Woman's Empowerment Coach and business mentor who helps women by having them face their fears and limiting beliefs that hinder then from living the life they dream of. Denise has a clear vision for seeing the trouble-spots that exist in, every "stuck" situation and the creativity to transform it instantly. She is a partner with YOUR OWN UNIVERSITY, best-selling author and the host of "It's YOUR Turn" Radio Show. Through her own struggles and divorce, Denise has managed to come out of it with a smiling face and a positive attitude through it all.

Denise's current mission is completing her book that will launch on Women's Day 2017. And she is the co-author of the book titled The Energy of Happiness that launched Jan. 28, 2015 and went straight to Amazons Best Seller within hours of the launch.

When Denise is not coaching women she is enjoying family time, cooking, traveling and going to rock concerts.

Learn more about Denise at http://www.denisedominguez. com and join the fun and wisdom at https://www.facebook/

pages/denise-dominguez

http://denisedominguez.com/self-love-training

CHAPTER 17

Choosing Life

Susan Ball

Now That You're My Wife...

It was a whirlwind romance. The kind where you're swept off your feet and left breathless. He was handsome, rugged, and passionate. He was good with my daughters. He took them out so I could have a break. He would drive me to work on a cold winter day and tell me how he loved taking care of us, and doing the little extras.

He bought me and my beautiful daughters a big Victorian house with a backyard. The house was in a lovely small town just two hours away from family and friends. He told me how he wanted the girls to have a place to invite friends and play freely.

I fell deeply, madly in love.

He pushed to get married and I thought why not. We had been together for over a year and marriage seemed a natural step.

He chose my birthday weekend as the date and told me how

we would spend romantic weekends celebrating our anniversary and my birthday. Sigh - he had me.

We wed. Small gathering and a nice party. Wedding night at the Royal York Hotel in downtown Toronto. It's a 5-star hotel and very posh. I was being pampered.

The morning after we were on our way to our short honeymoon in Niagara Falls. He reached to grab my hand and of course I responded with affection. But something was very different. He was squeezing my hand very hard and he said to me:

> *"Now that you are my wife, you will do as you're told, how you're told and when you're told."*

Initially I thought he was joking. I was wrong, very wrong. The man was a brutal fraud. My life turned into a living hell and I had been married one-day!

I married in October and I was running for my life to the police station in January. I moved out in February. The marriage lasted four short months and in that time I was strangled to blacking out, raped, emotionally abused, cheated on, and ridiculed in public.

After the worst beating, I lay on the floor and I decided right there and then that it was time to leave. I could not and would not let my young daughters watch their mother being abused. What kind of example was that setting?

I had no money, no job, no car or license but I had determination. I called friends and family. All but one said no I couldn't stay with them. They were very sorry for what I was going through but were unable to help.

My cousin came through and we moved into her furnace room in the basement. And in that dark, lonely furnace room is where I got stuck in my victim story and I started to abuse alcohol, drugs and men. I fell deeply into the well of victim'hood and I used it as crutch.

Rage and Weep

Drunk and singing Somewhere Over the Rainbow was a moment. Not necessarily the moment but one where I realized that I had reached rock bottom.

I was living in my cousin's furnace room. My bed was literally tucked in beside the furnace. From a 5-bedroom house to a furnace room was quite a tumble. I chose alcohol, drugs and nasty boys as a way to escape.

It was an avoidance tactic. I was avoiding facing and leaning into my emotions. If you're drunk, you can't feel. If you're drunk, you don't think about reality. If you're chasing bad boys, you feel vindicated and at some strange level, loved.

I went to my group counselling where we talked about him and evaluated all the reasons why he might be an abusive jerk. Everyone told their stories of pain and lost love and we celebrated being victims of our abusers.

Not once did we talk about how we were healing our wounds. How we were stepping out of our fear and into our power as free women. We didn't talk about self-love, or authenticity, or gratitude.

I would leave and go party not realizing I was covering up and burying the deep emotional pain that I had. Instead of letting it bubble up to the surface and release, I would suppress through alcohol and negative, self-destructive behaviour.

Over the Rainbow seemed so far away. I believed somewhere didn't exist for me. Why not? Because I was stuck in my Victim Story.

I had not allowed myself time to Rage and Weep. To mourn at

my deepest level. I put on my victim and I used it as the greatest excuse to fail at the rest of my life.

Your story is the greatest obstacle to your success.

Your story is so much more than what "happened" to you. I got all caught up in my victim story. It was comfortable there. I could talk about it. I could let it comfort me. I could let it determine how I acted. My life made sense.I hung onto my story because I was afraid to let it go. Letting it go felt like I would fall into a dark abyss filled with nothing and no-one. I was terrified of the emptiness that I thought would be the result of letting my story go.

You keep your story because it's safe. As long as you tell that story, you don't have to step out of your comfort zone and *face your fears*. It's easy to get stuck and it takes a great deal of courage to get un-stuck. It takes dedication, determination and desire to live with freedom, peace and happiness.

When I did decide to let my victim story go and let go of the past hurts, I walked into my greatest story. One that keeps growing and improving.

I realized that my story had taught me so much about what I wanted in my life. What was acceptable and who I would embrace on my new journey.

Consciously deciding to let my past go was the most terrifying and rewarding experience rolled together! I am so happy I stepped out of my past, healed and stepped into my brilliant present.

Recognizing and *accepting* that your abusive relationship was a fraud and that you are not responsible for what happened is a key step to letting go of your victim story.

Your Prince was a Toad

There were signs that the man was an abuser. What I thought was romantic, kind, considerate and caring were actually the steps he took to isolate me and my children.

Signs Your Romantic Prince may be an Abusive Toad:

- Isolation from family and friends. He bought me a house but it was two-hours away from my family. I didn't drive at the time so I became very dependent on him.

- He went to my employer and quit my job for me. He said we were fine without the money and the girls needed me at home. What he really did was make me Financially Dependent.

- Odd Moments of Ridicule. Going out for the evening and being told that he would be proud of me if I wore something that he personally chose. Usually, it was an inappropriate outfit and I would feel embarrassed and my confidence would plummet.

- Correcting me in public. Always. I lost my voice.

- Stopping my personal growth. I wanted to drive. I wanted to go to university. I was ridiculed for thinking that someone like me could do either.

- Sexual demands. Threats of having an affair if I didn't comply.

- No public displays of affection.

In retrospect, it was all there. I wasn't aware because I wanted to believe in the relationship and him. I wanted the dream he was selling. I didn't sign up for the nightmare he delivered.

I lacked self-confidence and he fed on that. He was able to manipulate me and my emotions. He was the problem, not you.

Your Journey to Rebel Thriver Begins with G.R.A.C.E.

I was done with pitying myself and playing the victim. Even though I'd been through the fires of an abusive relationship, I decided to not allow that toxicity to define my future.

I was ready to let go of my victim story and begin to create my fearless, vibrant, successful story.

But I didn't know how.

I felt stuck within a mess of my own negative labels and limiting beliefs. I knew I was hidden deep down under the pile of labels I'd acquired, I just had to uncover her again.

I longed for the me that was free and confident and felt equipped to tackle anything she set her mind to. I missed her! I wanted to find her again and live her and be her.

I learned that the first and best way to move on is to start by loving yourself and your life again. Quite honestly, once I learned some strategies to get past my own self-judgment and let go of all the negative beliefs and labels, the opportunities to create big, bold, fearless new chapters were endless!

I am well now and I have forgiven myself and him and moved on.

If you have left toxic-emotionally abusive relationship, you can do the same. Letting go, moving on and embracing your big, bold next chapter is a series of small steps but the journey is worth it. Scary but worth it.

I know, I did it. And you can too. Let's get started.

G.R.A.C.E.

The 5 Key Steps to Thrive! & Love Your Life after Abuse are:

Gratitude | Release | Authenticity | Challenge | Embrace

I affectionately call the 5-Steps G.R.A.C.E. and you can practice G.R.A.C.E. anytime, anywhere and with anyone. Commit to embracing your future happiness. Choose to Rebel against your victim story!

Practice G.R.A.C.E. and you will get where you want to go! You will notice shifts in your emotional, physical, and spiritual wellbeing.

Gratitude – What Am I Grateful For?

There is always something to be grateful for. The smallest of things bring me the greatest gratitude.

When you feel you are "stuck" in your darkest moment, gratitude will provide the way out. During dark times, it's hard to see positive forces when obstacles are blaring and fears are looming.

Gratitude shifts your mind to focus on the good and positive things that are happening. Start small and be grateful for your breath, your health, your children, the sun, the $5 you have in your wallet.

Each time you purposefully find gratitude in a negative situation, you shift your mindset. And that begins your healing journey.

Release: What Can I Release? Let Go?

I bet you're holding on to all kinds of negative junk. The junk you're holding on to is cluttering your mind and your path forward. Yeah, that's the truth!

The things you hold on to, bear grudges or perhaps feel angry and hurt about cloud your mind and prevent you from being the best you can be.

They are baggage. Heavy, overloaded baggage. The kind you would pay extra for when you travel. And the kind you are paying a hefty price for right now!

I was holding on to junk that had been handed to me during a violent relationship.

I had bags containing anger - at him, at me, at people who should have rescued me.

I had bags containing guilt - my children saw some of the bad stuff, my family warned me and I didn't listen and these bags led to new bags filled with: Anger!

For me, I was hanging on to my victim story because it was safe. As a victim, I had no responsibility for my actions. I didn't have to look at my life and make the changes I needed to move forward. It was comfortable and safe.

What did I need to let go of? – my victim story

How did I benefit from holding on? – comfort, no responsibility, fear of the future

Authentic Me: Who the Hell Am I Anyway?

Through life's experiences, the opinion of others, and the abusive situation, I had buried my authenticity under piles of rubbish. There was all of the stuff I had been programmed to believe I couldn't do. There was the negative stuff that I had attached to my self-image. There was a fear and disbelief that I would never find me again.

But I did and I'm amaZing.
You Can Find Your Authentic Self Too!

So where do you find this authentic self? It's hiding under layers of protection and conditioning and to find you, you want to gradually strip away those layers. It's a process that begins with questions.

What do I love to do? What makes me smile? What am I doing

that makes me irritable? Or feel stress?

Find the things you love to do. Hang out with people who let you be you. Let go of things and people who make you feel uncomfortable or stressed.

Challenge: What is My Next Challenge?

Challenges are everywhere in your life. It's not the challenge that will keep you stuck, it's how you handle it. And the best way to handle challenges is to get out in front of them.

Challenges are overcome when they are changed to goals with an action plan. When we look at any challenge and ask "what do I need to do to change this?", we immediately set a course of action that we are going to take. You can't change the outcome if you continue to do the same thing.

Challenges require Change and Change is Growth.

Embrace: What Can I Embrace as Possible?

When we leave an abusive relationship, we are caught in "impossibilities". All the I cant's come to the surface and keep us stuck.

Moving from your "impossibilities" to all the amazing possibilities that are waiting for you, happens with Positive Affirmations. They are all about awakening your potential so you can see your infinite possibilities. They reaffirm all that you can do. All that you are and all that you can be.

Every time you write or say your affirmation, you are reinforcing your new positive belief and overwriting your old negative one.

Start your affirmations with I am, I can or I will.

I am successful. I can move forward. I will build a life that I love.

ABOUT THE AUTHOR

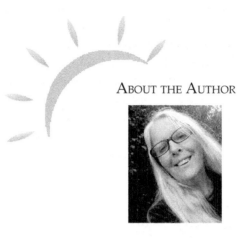

Susan Ball

Susan is a skilled and experienced Women's Freedom Coach, Self-Love Activist, and the creator of Rebel Thriver, a 4-Step Healing Process to Love Your Life Again After an Abusive Relationship, as well as being a survivor of an abusive relationship herself.

Through her Rebel Thriver programs, Susan motivates and guides her clients to restore confidence, balance, wellbeing, and joy. To fall, deeply, madly in love with themselves so they can live fulfilling and confident lives and fully embrace big, bold, blissful living.

She brings this intuition along with proven strategies to her work, much to her clients' delight. She works with women who are ready to transition into their power, passion, and purpose.

The result is that they can attract the right people into their life, experience increased confidence to say no without feeling guilty and create an identity that is not tied to a past negative experience.

Susan is a regular contributor to It's Your Turn Radio, Huffington Post, and dreams of living off the grid in her 'Tiny Wrecky House'.

For additional resources and inspiration, stay connected to Susan through her website: www.susanball.ca; Facebook; and Twitter.

CHAPTER 18

Creating the Wait

Karey Keith

When you want to make changes in your life, such as leaving an abusive relationship, making a career change, or moving to another location, you often have to wait for life's circumstances to catch up with your desired action. This waiting time is not the time to sit around and worry, or otherwise ruminate on your fears. Instead, you can take this time and use it productively and powerfully for your own benefit. I call it "Creating the Wait."

Creating the Wait is a valuable skill for all areas of life. It is an attitude of hope and love that empowers our voice and enables our future to bloom and grow. It is also a time of trusting ourselves in a way that is personal and liberating. Every person that I have ever coached in mastering a wait has come out the other side grounded and self-assured. Often the outcomes are different than expected as we move out of codependency into self-awareness. This process and how you create your wait is personal and varies per situation. It is vital in leaving abusive situations.

When leaving abuse, the wait falls into three main categories, acute, chronic and mundane. Each of these requires different timing and strategy, but all are worth the effort as the outcomes are tremendously empowering. Let's face it, when in the hell of abuse, we feel forced to give up our power in self-defense as that is how the abuser controls us.

In the acute situation, we know the abusers are mean and we are the victims. However, you cannot heal from a place of victimhood, as it is void of power. In a chronic abusive relationship, the abuse is harder to recognize as the abuser beats you down then picks you up. The same person who comforts you when you are down is the one who beat you down in the first place. This type of abuse is confusing, hard to leave, and keeps us controlled in a seemingly loving way, but it is a lie and an energetic pattern that we must understand to escape.

The chronic situation is more emotional or psychological than physical. In fact, the abuser can appear to be a perfect fit for us. The abuser is actually controlling us by manipulating our thought patterns and responding in what might be a passive aggressive manner. This type of abuse is difficult to leave because it is often so difficult to recognize.

The mundane situation is when we know who the abuser is and who we are, but the situation is tolerable enough to wait for the kids to graduate, money to come, etc. In this choice to wait, it is important to create the wait vs. falling into complacency. Complacency has little power to drive the ultimate change.

Most abusers feed on taking our power. We justify giving them our power because we love them, we need the security, or perhaps we just don't know any better. Abuse is NOT love, period. Twisting it up to be love is a lie. In particular, I don't know any woman on the planet that has completely escaped this lesson. Love is the creative force. Love is the supportive force. As humans, we are the blend of creative and supportive love. Creative love comes direct from the creative force, and supportive love comes from Mother Earth. We are the love and it grows from within. If you are not happy, or do not know that you ARE the love, then let us explore how creating a wait allows you to remedy that non-truth.

Why create a wait when leaving abuse?

The number one reason is self-defense. Abuse hurts us on all levels and distorts our sense of self. Like it or not, we allow this dynamic and it is hard to undo. Creating a wait allows us to gather strength and vitality and formulate a strategy. It also gives space for healing, self-discovery, and truth to prevail. In acute abuse, often the fight or flight response causes us to leave first. However, without an immediate strategy for recovery by designing a waiting place to heal and regroup, the abused often go back to the abuser over and over, choose this type of partner again, or remain victim forever. In acute abuse, the wait is essential for healing, grieving, and regaining power along with self-worth. This is also true in chronic abuse but the timing and strategy are different.

When do we create a wait while leaving abuse?

In acute abuse it times out in two ways. They hurt you or yours so you pack essentials, leave, and immediately create the wait, often in stages. Or, the abuser destroys trust in an intense way, but you want your stuff and the clean escape, which requires quick strategy into a safe wait. Either way it is nothing short of traumatic. Either way we must grab the wait as our safe place and keep moving towards the new. Setting the new and healing the old is essential in creating happiness. You deserve to be happy. Happiness is created by your conscious choices, always. Own this fact.

Escaping chronic abuse is most efficiently done with a wait before you go. Often the abuse is psychological and/or passive aggressive and you feel confused. If you are confused as to whether the problems are your fault or not, it is essential that you bring into awareness your energy patterns, habits, beliefs, coping patterns, and reactions. It is important that you understand your codependence patterns; what they are and how they contribute to your reality before you try to change your reality. This wait before you go allows safety, healing and opens the window of hope towards the new adventures in life. If you don't reset yourself before you go, more often than not, you return or attract the same lessons again. This wait is a special opportunity to create the new, heal the present and past while regaining vitality and clarity. You are clear in what you don't want. It is imperative that you get clear on what you do want "for you" vs. waiting for other people to change allowing you to be happy. You are in charge of happy, make that choice. Sometimes you have to create a wait after you leave too, especially if you have never lived alone. You can plant the next phase of life like a beautiful garden while you heal, plan, and move through the hell of the change. Doing all these phases at once not only distracts you from the pain of it all, but shortens the full recovery time by half.

Mundane abuse often takes the form of neglect. Chronic neglect is abuse. When it turns into mundane, complacency is the outcome. With this type of abuse we often are so used to it that we do not fight it anymore. Acceptance is a good but what we often do not realize with this type of abuse is that we are already in a wait. A permanent, stagnant wait for other people and circumstance to change is the outcome of our choice to be complacent. Mental abuse, alcohol overuse, etc. can fall in this category as we adhere to "in sickness and in health" or other justifications for living with uncooperative people.

We often see this in long-term relationships who partner in parenting. I left my husband in 2003 with two small boys. It was hard. The abuse went from chronic to acute back to chronic and then hit a plateau of mundane for years before my boys were deemed old enough to move away by the courts. When the youngest turned 14, I had been complacent for so long that I was not sure leaving was best.

How do you motivate yourself for change when you have accepted less than what everyone deserves? You go deep and wide to find your truth. My truth that I should be free of the misery of other people's choices was strong. It was a hidden ember that I found and nurtured back to life. Find the ember of the truth that you are. Nurture it and turn the flame into a passion for living again. Your passion, your life by design, is what fuels you to turn that wait into a springboard for happy living.

How do you create a wait?

In all circumstances, you create your wait as a safe place to allow growth and healing. In this feeling of safety, you can learn to trust yourself, your guides, Masters, human and animal support teams. You are never alone. You have others. Even if all you think you have is a guardian angel or your dog – that is enough. You can learn to access and use the guides, angels and Masters at your will. The animals, flora and fauna alike, are there for us too. Open up to all the love around you.

So, step one of the process is to create a safe place to access your truth and draw from your support team. Step two is to evaluate what you dream of vs. what you are living. And step three is to plan the new and start healing from the old. I know this sounds easier than it feels when in the drama of things. However, starting is as easy as this effective exercise.

1. While seated, allow your energy to go deep into the Earth. Deep in the Earth is an extra dimension of pure supportive love. Tap into that dimension and bring the pure supportive love back up into our body. Fill your

body with pure supportive love.

2. Now send your energy past the clouds, angels and Masters, shapes, colors, and tones of your life until you reach pure creative love. Bring the love of creation back down into your body. Fill your body with creative love.

3. Synergize the creative and supportive love in perfect balance in your body. Feel the balance.

4. Hold out your hands and create a ball of light. In the ball of light, you can intend anything you choose. (Intentions like "show me my truth," "fill me with courage and strength," or "send money for the move" are all easy to start with.) Fill the ball of light with your intention.

5. Call in Archangel Michael, the blue light, Jesus, Buddha, Goddess, Creator or any high frequency that you trust, and hand off your ball of light to your trusted Spirit.

Your intentions and trust will build with this exercise. Do it often. Keep yourself balanced.

There are many tools and techniques to help you move back into happiness. Creating your wait will quietly allow you to heal while you empower your greatest dreams, plan and execute your changes, and learn the truth that life is yours to design. You are the love. Taking back your power for life is exercising free will, your free will. You are the wisdom. Love Wisdom is the lesson of the Christ and the balance you can learn through a wait you created and executed through your free will can bring you to happy and give you peace.

About the Author

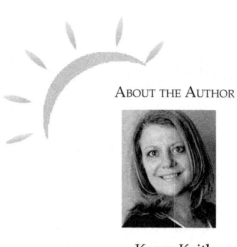

Karey Keith

Karey is a psychic medium, relationship coach, teacher, and healer. She specializes in helping people move out of stagnant life circumstances and into vibrant living. Her approach is honest, empowering, and effective.

Karey has been working as a psychic for more than 20 years. She began her spiritual practice at the age of seven by spontaneously channeling the Masters.

Helping people find their personal truth through a soul perspective is Karey's life calling. Trained in multiple healing modalities, equips Karey with many tools, tips, and perspectives. She is ready and able to help you design your life through conscious choice. Her intuitive accuracy and honest, down-to-earth perspectives can quickly get to the root of your issues.

She is a loving mother of three boys and lives in the North West USA.

Website: http://majesticinsights.com

Facebook: https://www.facebook.com/majestic.insights

Email: majesticinsights@gmail.com

CHAPTER 19

Never Enough...The Lie of a Lifetime

Becky Herdt

There it was... after over 25 plus years of my adult life spent looking for a way to get past all of the limitations and stories of my past... being coached, and trained, and guided, and sponsored along the way... I found myself looking deep into the eyes of an amazing friend. "Wow," he said softly, somewhat surprised. "It all comes back to that thing of not being enough, doesn't it?" There was no judgment or harshness in his words, only kindness. A kindness accompanied by the recognition of the frightened child in front of him, who was terrified of letting anyone in.

"What if you were to, for even twenty seconds, see you through my eyes? The way I see you? Can you do that?" he continued. And in the moments that followed, it all came flooding in.

I could perceive the energy of what he saw when he looked at me, and the most bizarre things started to show up. I really could see me through the eyes of a friend. Not just in those twenty seconds, but ongoing. I could feel and see the energies of kindness (*my* kindness) staring back at me. The energy of my potencies, my capacities, and my brilliances. I say the energy of these things, as I didn't really have a picture of what those things were...and I didn't suddenly get a download of my laundry list of brilliance. I couldn't necessarily see tangible examples in that moment. I just knew that "yes...that *is* me." (It seems important to clarify here that "brilliance" is not about intellectual abilities, or being smart. True brilliance is the light of who I truly *be*, not what I *do*...it's the magic and uniqueness of me, how I see the world and what I have to contribute to this planet and mankind).

A jumping off place was right in front of me – a moment of truth. Was I willing to actually receive this kindness and see what else was truly possible? Or would I resort to one of my trusted standbys to deflect it? Whirling before me, a thousand images rolled through my mind – my entire history of places and spaces where I had trusted people (individuals and groups, including family, religious and social acquaintances) and subsequently been hurt, betrayed, used. Many people had labeled these past scenarios as abuse and I could acknowledge the threads of truth in that. And yet I consistently resisted the idea– it sounded so pathetic. Did I really need to have someone to blame for all the places I wasn't perfect? At the same time "survivor" never quite felt like me either.

I created a polarity around the abuse – I either resisted any identity with it, or I allowed myself to be enveloped in the victimization. I couldn't find the middle ground and wasn't asking any questions. I was simply stuck in a reactionary pattern of self-loathing. I put on a happy face and avoided the conversations and the need to really look at these life events by using the excuse that I didn't wish to be defined or limited by the stories of my past. When push came to shove, I would acknowledge the abuse with a few words, and then talk about how I had forgiven people, and I would move on. I used it as part of my "story" in a very controlled way... where it suited me and to get people to stop talking to me about it! And I would never, ever really be with the energy of it and acknowledge how much I had been hurt or what had been taken from me. All the while, I would agree with the adage that it's 'All Good' and try to look at "What's right about this that I'm not getting?" And every time I would ask myself that question, I would go into judgment about me and the pathetic creation of my life. I understood such questions were designed to help me have awareness, and yet it seemed to only put me into a space of the wrongness of me (after all, who would choose this?) and reignite the cycle of feeling like I was never enough.

All the while, I somehow knew that it wasn't about me doing anything to deserve it... that the sexual acts of older relatives thrust upon me, beginning when I was a small child, were not ok. I knew that when I finally decided to tell what had happened, and I was met with words from spiritual "leaders" like "boys will be boys and it's the girls responsibility to say no to sexual advances" and "surely you know better than that – why didn't you say something?" that those words were not okay. And yet, despite the fact that so many of the things said to me under the umbrella of "love" and "spirituality" were actually things that kept me stuck in the limitations and smallness of me, I somehow bought the lie that I was responsible for it all, that I was somehow lacking, that I wasn't enough, that 'if only...' There were so, so many if only's.

The real twisted place is that even when people truly loved me with no distortion, it was very hard if not impossible for me to receive it and/or trust it. I had learned early and learned well that I could smile and nod and still be on hyper alert. Not that the state of alert allowed me to avoid the abuse, but it somehow made me feel like I had more control of my world. At least I could perceive it was coming and prepare myself. And then the next step of the evolution was just expecting it. Like somehow it was just part of what I came to this planet to do. The elusive feeling of control was such a lie…and it certainly didn't include allowing me to be vulnerable with anyone. It didn't include looking at the places and spaces where I was amazing. Nor did it include being willing to totally let my barriers and let someone in. Heaven forbid! It only allowed for me to stay stuck in the lie of not being enough and somehow being responsible for all of the behaviors and beliefs of everyone around me.

In recent years, I had received similar invitations before to step into a different reality, to see myself through someone else's eyes and sometimes I would take tentative steps towards it. But for whatever reason, I had never been able to fully choose it, to fully choose me. All while knowing on some level that no matter what happened, no matter what other people did or didn't do…I would be ok. And I had decided I could be content, even if never happy. Happiness, after all, was entirely overrated. It seemed like a fleeting whim, rather than a choice. I somewhere decided that I should instead settle for some happy moments along the way.

Unkindness and limitations were so much more familiar, and I knew how to dance with those. Through years of practice, I was quite skilled at keeping people at arm's length. My life was a stage and I was a brilliant actor…bringing people in just close enough so that I didn't have to live in a vacuum. All the while never really letting them in, never letting them see all of me. The only parts visible were those I chose to expose. It was all just a case of 'managing the audience.' I was willing to be somewhat vulnerable to most of them. Although usually when they started getting too close, I'd find a way to cut that off before I could get hurt. The old adage of "keep your friends close and your enemies closer" took on a life of its own in my world and I never made it easy for people to be there for me. Everyone was a potential danger. Even when I would open up to pieces and parts of my world, all the while making them think they knew me well. I always somehow knew I would be ok, no matter what happened. At the same time, the true kindness of others, especially men, was never easy for me to receive. It scared me and left me suspicious of what might follow. And I usually chose a way to deflect any such kindness with (often self-deprecating) humor.

And there was the mirror for me to see it... I was continuing to buy the belief, the judgment, the lie that I wasn't enough. No matter how much my brilliance appeared to others, or how much they could see my kindness, my potency to change things, my business brilliance (and yes, I suppose the list does go on and on if I were but to look for it). I never trusted that I was really any of those things, much less all of them. Sometimes I could see glimpses of it (usually when there was some herculean outcome or when I received praise from others about something I had done or accomplished). And sometimes I could perceive the kindness that was so much who I "be" that I either discounted it or took it for granted. All of the glimpses and pieces over time were somehow never enough. Me, truly being me, was never enough. Or so I thought.

My life, like that of many others I knew, had consisted of moments of fun and laughter, mixed in with moments of intensity and wishing to no longer be on this planet. I considered myself lucky to have lots of humor around me when I was growing up. It wasn't until years later that I realized how much I used that humor (in myself and others) as a soft weapon, deflecting the things that hit close to home and as a way of keeping people at arm's length, all while making them feel like they knew me. With this barrier of humor, I could keep people out and I didn't have to be vulnerable. I could protect myself from being hurt. My sense of humor was, in and of itself, a brilliant creation.

In the weeks that followed and up until this very moment, more and more "aha!" moments have begun to unfold. My willingness to see myself through the eyes of a friend began to shift and change the way I saw myself. It wasn't the first time I had seen myself through someone else's eyes... it was just the first time that the someone was someone who actually admired, respected, cared for me. I had made one of my life habits seeing myself through the eyes of others. The difference is that all the ways I had done that in the past – somehow it never included people that actually liked me. It certainly included family members, colleagues, and people that were in my social and religious circles. But these people didn't actually like me. And the energetic sponge I was, I picked up every nuance of judgment, every hint of wrongness, every sliver of them being superior (knowing more, being smarter, more clever, or even more able to control others) And perhaps more importantly, often times people who didn't actually seem to like themselves – and I picked up on that. I was always very intuitive and very good at reading people. However, I later discovered that the things I believed about me were actually things that I picked up from people who thought very little of me. The line between their energy and mine had become so blurred that I couldn't distinguish between the two!

I started looking at all of this through the eyes of one of the basic tools of Access Consciousness.... Who Does This Belong To? It speaks to the concept that most of us are little energetic sponges that go around soaking up all the thoughts, ideas, beliefs, judgments, emotions of others. Freedom really comes when we return to sender all the things that aren't ours. And when I still felt weird and out of sorts with the energies arising, or the judgments and doubts, I'd use another tool of a similar vein: "Who Am I Being?" So, for all the ways I am thinking, behaving, judging myself, being not enough and even pathetic – Who I am being when I am being that? Who was like that in my life? Wow! It wasn't really me at all! I was only mimicking the behavior and energies of others around me (both family and friends and fellow church-goers, not to mention a large number of people that live on this planet with me). If I were truly being me, what would my life really be like? Would I really believe that I am not enough and have never been enough? Would I really believe that lie of a lifetime? Again, wow! Who knew? Turns out when I am truly being me – I can tap into the magic of me… without the distortions of judging myself as not being enough. Who knew?!

The true resonance with the idea that *everything* in my life, up to and including that moment, was created by the choices I had made. It didn't mean I came here to be abused. It just meant that life was a series of interesting choices, and I could make myself wrong for it or I could just acknowledge where I was and move forward from there I would not allow myself to be identified as a victim – inexplicable and unfortunate things happening to me… at the mercy and design of others. And I could see myself as the gift and the magic that I truly am… just like I could see it and perceive it when I looked at me through the eyes of a true friend.

Everything in my life and my world has continued to change since that moment. I'm able to see and claim my gifts and capacities. And while I still occasionally, almost as if by reflex, go to the wrongness of me… I don't stay there long. I recognize it for what it is and I quickly choose beyond it. What if I never again had to buy into the lie of a lifetime? What if I trusted me more than anyone else, and could believe that the universe has my back? What if I always could know and remember that I am enough… more than enough…and that this world is lucky to have me in it? What if I can simply keep choosing to be me, and always know that's all that's required? Ahhh! Yes! I'll have that!

Thus the leap of faith was launched. Choosing to be me. Choosing to not hide. Choosing to receive the judgment of any and every one. Choosing to be willing to lose everything. And with each of the choices, more space showed up. More ease. More sense of the possibilities.

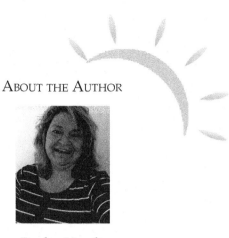

Becky Herdt

Becky Herdt, MBA, is an International Business and Success Coach, Motivational Speaker, Radio Show Host of "Unchained with Becky", Best-selling author, Right Relationship For You Certified Facilitator, and Access Consciousness Certified Facilitator. Becky brings her vast experience in multi-national business, elementary education, intuitive healing and human relationships/family dynamics to facilitate people who are ready to choose beyond the reality that they currently are experiencing.

Is now the time to dig deep and yet keep quickly moving beyond the stickiness, beyond the story, to exponentialize the possibilities in your life and living, contact becky@beckyherdt.com. What if your life is truly about choice? What if you could find your life and laughter? Are you ready to be free to be and choose you? What if you are the gift and the change that the world requires? What can we create together for you, and for the world?

For more information:
www.beckyherdt.com
www.unchainedwithbecky.com
www.beckyherdt.accessconsciousness.com
http://rightrelationshipforyou.com/profile/Becky-Herdt/

CHAPTER 20

From Survival to Thrival

Minette the Energist

Life is Amazing!! Successful business doing what I LOVE, Amazing family and a life filled with joy and possibilities. How does it get any better than that?!?

Although this was not always so, it has been quite a journey to get here. Like so many I have survived many forms of abuse (physical, mental, emotional and so on). I am a Survivor and this made me very proud and sad at the same time. It seemed I still also carried shame and anger. However, me being a survivor gave me strength, I had overcome and SURVIVED! What better feeling is there than that?

Unfortunately, that's the way I was living my life, in Survival Mode. I found myself creating my life from my story. I was clinging to it and repeatedly playing it over and over. I was choosing to (at the time not realizing that it was a choice) continually create my own suffering by carrying my heavy story. It had mentally, emotionally, physically and spiritually penetrated every cell in my body. I used it to create the form and structure of my life. I always felt like if people knew what I had lived through, then and only then, could they truly understand me. I started using my story as a connection point to relate to others and where they were in their life or justify where I was in mine. I mean, how could someone who had been through what I had been through ever live a normal happy life?

For those of you who are or have ever lived in survival mode, you know it is a different way to function. It affects not only you but those of everyone around you. I had very little patience for people. I was always looking for order and stability. Even laughter would bother me; What are they laughing at? Don't they realize all the terrible things happening in the world? If they had experienced what I had they would not have joy either? I was living a smaller life and the majority of my decisions were based out of fear. The level of fear I carried was suffocating. I was afraid to love with all my heart because I did not want to ever let anyone have the power to hurt me again. I was limiting my relationships with other people because in survivor mode, I could trust no one but myself. I had seen what other people could do and how cruel they can be, even those closest to you. You learn to rely solely on yourself. This for me was a very empowering and sad way of choosing to live life. I had, what I know now to be the illusion of control over my life. But no one to truly share it with (including myself). Because I was living a life in Survival Mode and not Thrival Mode.

What had I made so vital about hoarding these traumatic memories that kept me functioning in Survivor Mode?

I had made my story so significant, because I just wanted someone to understand. I soon figured out that expecting someone to understand my story and exactly what I had been through was not going to happen. Even if they were raised in the same family, their point of view was different. Because everyone's story and point of view is different. So waiting for someone to come along truly get me and understand what I had been through was not going to happen. As soon as I acknowledged this, I was able to start to letting the significance of my story go. What had I made so important about others knowing my story? Was this vital to my healing or creating a life I truly desire? Would their confirmation and acknowledgment of how terrible it was bring me comfort? I knew it was terrible, and I stopped making it vital that others understood how terrible it was? This was very freeing as it allowed me to start to choose something different. This helped me realize something that was key to my healing. Everyone has experienced some sort of pain in their lives, they all had their own stories. When I stopped comparing stories or using them to gauge people and their lives, my life started to change, because I finally stopped judging my life/story. It allowed me to realize that while we all have pain, we choose how long we suffer. Being free from my story allowed me to stop suffering. It was not overnight, but day by day and step by step my journey to healing from the abuse began.

Mental Healing

I saw others choose to stay a victim, always functioning from fear, blaming others for what was happening in their life, always waiting for the next fist to strike or the next terrible thing to happen. I saw how this decision not only affected them but everyone around them. I wanted my life to be different, I wanted more for the next generation. So, I decided that I would take control over my life and stop being a victim. Healing mentally seemed to be, for me, the first logical step as I could not quiet my mind. I was literally thinking myself crazy. I, like so many others, wanted to understand: Why did this happen to me? How could they do this to me? How could people be so cruel? I went down so many paths trying to figure this out. I studied Psychology, joined groups, started counseling and became a counselor. I spent so much time and energy on these questions, as if the answers would somehow make it all OK or lessen the pain. I came to the conclusion that, there were no real answers, just what I consider today "Choices". For whatever reason this did happen to me and they did these terrible things, it was a choice. Yes, there is their circumstances, they came from abusive households, that's what their generation was like, they had suffered violence and atrocities too. But not everyone that has these experiences repeats these actions or continues the cycle. It is a choice. So I made a choice that I would be the one to break the cycle of violence. I would not use my background as an excuse to continue yet another generation of violence. I let go of my search for answers. When I let go, I realized that my quest for answers had been prolonging my suffering and I started to have a more peaceful mind.

Emotional Healing

With a more peaceful mind I noticed I was still suffering, just not as much. My thoughts had quieted, which was great. With this quieter mind I started to have a greater awareness of my emotions. Thus began the emotional healing part of my journey. This is where I allowed myself to be vulnerable. Which is something I had never let myself do before (survivors are not vulnerable, being vulnerable is a weakness). This opinion quickly changed when I realized just how much pain the emotions I had bottled up inside were causing. It felt like this intense storm, a volcano that I never knew when or where would erupt. Because while I had quieted my mind from the questions and accepted my circumstances in my mental healing, I had suffocated my heart and took the attitude of suck it up and be grateful for where you are now. It could always be worse. These were the type of things I told myself daily. I never acknowledged the fear, anger, rage, sadness, betrayal, hurt and so many other emotions I had shoved down to be strong and survive. This choice seemed to leave me in a constant state of anxiety and worry. For those of you who have ever lived like this, you know you can hardly call it living. It is a constant state of anguish and despair. I felt lost and alone. At my lowest point one day I decided this was not working for me anymore. I was desiring to start creating a life worth living. I was ready for happiness and joy. So I decided to acknowledge and allow my feelings to come out. I asked questions when a feeling arose. This is an example of that dialogue:

What is this I am feeling?
Anger

Why am I angry?
Because the people who were supposed to protect me, are the ones who hurt me most. Because I was not strong enough to stop the abuse.

Is holding onto this anger helping or hurting me?
Hurting

Am I ready to let it go?
Yes

I repeated this sort of dialogue with ever emotion that arose, I was vulnerable to all my feelings and acknowledged them. It was miraculous for me how by just acknowledging these feelings how quickly the energy/pain started to dissipate. It was like my heart started to become light and smile, for the first time. Happiness started to creep back into my life. I started to feel better and have a more peaceful and joyful heart.

Life was definitely getting better, my relationships improved and I was starting to enjoy life. But for some reason, I seemed to be chronically ill. Then came the next step of my healing journey. I had the awareness that my body required healing too.

Physical Healing

Though my body appeared physically healed, there were no longer any bruises, my wounds had healed and left scars. There was this energy present, almost trapped. It was then I knew that the abuse had permeated my cells and left almost a residue in my body. I came to realize, while the abuse was taking place there were times I would leave my body and kind of "Check Out". When I had this realization, I came to understand that no amount of mental processing or positive attitude would address this next layer of physical healing that my body required.

I started by being present with my body in a way I never had before, sensing where there was a density/pain or energy. I began talking to my body as a conscious being, a best friend, acknowledging the pain it had endured and expressing my gratitude for the strong body that it is. I let my body know that I appreciated what a great contribution it was and remained to me. I let my body know, that I knew what it had been through and that whatever dis-comfort/dis- ease it was creating to protect me was no longer required. I let my body know it was safe. This acknowledgment and reassurance of safety seemed to change the energy of my entire body. This was another huge step in my healing journey as it allowed my body to release energies it had carried for so long. This allowed by body to begin healing. So now with a peaceful mind, joyful heart and healing body, I finally felt like I had completed my healing journey. I was living a happy life. Until....

Spiritual Healing

My final step in my healing journey, came when someone told me everything that happens to us in life "we choose". This rocked my world. I was very confused and upset. Why would I have chosen this? How could a child choose this? It made no sense. I was living a happy life now, so I was able to reflect upon this in a different matter. I had conversations with people, it seemed many people especially in the spiritual world had this belief. I was told that when we truly accept everything that we chose and not only accept it but embrace it, as a contribution to where we are today, then our soul is free and has learned the lesson it chose to learn in this lifetime. Then our spirit can soar and our passion ignite as we become the contribution we are able to be in this lifetime. Being the invitation and inspiration for others to know it is possible. Something about this resonated with me. I had never thought about being an inspiration to others. I always desired to help people, but never thought to inspire. I had up until this time processed and released these heavy energies from my mind, heart and body. But never thought about my spirit or living a life with passion. I then said one of the hardest things I have ever said in my life, "I am grateful for everything that has happened to me in my life because I know it has lead to me being here now." I repeated this until I not only was saying the words but feeling the energy this created within me. I felt so much lighter, I felt changed. I felt inspired. It is so interesting the way the universe works.

The next day I came across another who was looking to heal. I shared with this person my story for the first time with no charge, there was no anger or sadness. It was just a series of events that no longer had a hold on me. I was not functioning from them, I was creating with them in a way I never had before, with gratitude. My sharing these events with this person in the way I did, brought her to tears. She said I had given her hope that she too could heal from abuse. She became my first client. My spirit did soar that day in a way I never thought possible, I had found my passion. This renewed energy of my spirit has led me to where I am creating from today. I am beyond happy. I am THRIVING! I am the invitation for others to know it's possible to not only survive abuse, but it is possible to thrive after abuse. I know now that everything that happened to me led to this point and I am grateful for that. I am now helping people all over the world live a life worth living, creating the realities they truly desire and switch from Survival Mode to Thrival Mode.

When and if we choose healing, only we can choose for ourselves when we are ready.

So if you are ready here are the things that helped me, maybe they might help another:

1. *Quiet your mind. Be aware of your thoughts and what they are creating in your life.*

2. *Acknowledge and release all the emotions you have bottled up inside.*

3. *Acknowledge your body and everything it has been though and thank it. Let your body know it is safe. Tell your body to release all the energies/pain it has been carrying.*

4. *Find your passion.*

On A Personal Note: I wanted to share with you that by me choosing to truly heal on all these levels, I have contributed to creating the first generation in my family line free from violence. My marriage, children and business are thriving. I coach clients all over the world. I am the invitation to the next generation that anything is possible. How does it get any better than that?!!

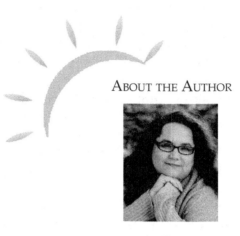

About the Author

Minette the Energist

My name is Minette Sanchez, also known as the Internal Energist. I am a certified professional life coach, energy worker, Access Consciousness® Certified Bars Practitioner and Facilitator as well as an Access Consciousness® Certified Body Process Facilitator, radio show host, motivational speaker, and author, with a background in business and psychology. I am the proud owner of Internal Energies, a company whose goal it is to help people create more ease, joy and possibilities in all aspects of their lives.

The End

CPSIA information can be obtained
at www.ICGtesting.com
Printed in the USA
BVOW04s2243041116
466993BV00011B/63/P